When Life Hands You Lemons, Make Lemon Meringue Pie

When Life Hands You Lemons, Make Lemon Meringue Pie

Seven Healing Recipes for Living
(and Thriving) with Cancer

JOANNA M. LUND

with *Barbara Alpert*

A PERIGEE BOOK

THE BERKLEY PUBLISHING GROUP
Published by the Penguin Group
Penguin Group (USA) Inc.
375 Hudson Street, New York, New York 10014, USA
Penguin Group (Canada), 90 Eglinton Avenue East, Suite 700, Toronto, Ontario M4P 2Y3, Canada
(a division of Pearson Penguin Canada Inc.)
Penguin Books Ltd., 80 Strand, London WC2R 0RL, England
Penguin Group Ireland, 25 St. Stephen's Green, Dublin 2, Ireland (a division of Penguin Books Ltd.)
Penguin Group (Australia), 250 Camberwell Road, Camberwell, Victoria 3124, Australia
(a division of Pearson Australia Group Pty. Ltd.)
Penguin Books India Pvt. Ltd., 11 Community Centre, Panchsheel Park, New Delhi—110 017, India
Penguin Group (NZ), cnr. Airborne and Rosedale Roads, Albany, Auckland 1310, New Zealand
(a division of Pearson New Zealand Ltd.)
Penguin Books (South Africa) (Pty.) Ltd., 24 Sturdee Avenue, Rosebank, Johannesburg 2196,
South Africa
Penguin Books Ltd., Registered Offices: 80 Strand, London WC2R 0RL, England

PRINTING HISTORY
Perigee trade paperback edition / October 2005

PERIGEE is a registered trademark of Penguin Group (USA) Inc.
The "P" design is a trademark belonging to Penguin Group (USA) Inc.

This book has been cataloged by the Library of Congress

PRINTED IN THE UNITED STATES OF AMERICA

10   9   8   7   6   5   4   3   2   1

Dedication

This book is dedicated in loving memory to my parents, Jerome and Agnes McAndrews. I feel the values they taught me as a child have helped me immensely while on my cancer journey—from "praying often" to "working hard."

This book is also dedicated to every person going through traumatic medical situations in their lives, including battling cancer.

And it is also dedicated to all the hardworking, caring medical professionals who treat cancer patients—from the doctors to the nurses to anyone else involved in cancer treatment.

I want to share with you the last poem my mother ever wrote—just days before she joined my father in Heaven. She knew her days here on Earth were numbered, but she still didn't question God—she simply trusted. Hopefully, her words will comfort you as much as they have me.

I Know

I know there is a God, because
  I feel His presence everywhere.
I know there is a God, for
  He has taken me in His care.

Sometimes, I doubt Him
  When I think my prayers go unheard.
Yet, I know He is aware of what
  I am praying for, every single word.

He answers in His own way
  According to His will.
So, I place my worries in His hands
  And tell my heart . . . be still.

Agnes Carrington McAndrews

Acknowledgments

While I cried often (did I ever mention that I'm extremely emotional?) while working on this book, many people handed me hankies, so to speak, so I could "see through my tears" and keep going.

For handing me those hankies, I want to thank:

Cliff Lund—my husband, and my helping hand while making this cancer journey. He did so much more than I ever expected! Cancer brought us even closer together. I'll never be able to thank him enough.

Barbara Alpert—my writing partner and friend. She's been involved in Race for the Cure for years and has been a helpful person to many. But when I asked her to help sort out my writings and feelings so others could make sense of them, I never dreamed she could do what she did! I'll be forever grateful for her help.

Coleen O'Shea—my literary agent. She often called just to

see how I was doing and to make sure I was resting when I should be. After I wrote several columns in my monthly food newsletter about my own cancer journey, she suggested I write even more and put them in a book. Without her, I might never have gone public with my personal story! I'm so glad she gave me that push.

John Duff—my publisher. He truly took a "leap of faith" when I shared that I wanted to write a book without recipes— after all, I've written more than thirty cookbooks for him. Yes, the title includes a reference to recipes, but that's all this book has in common with my cookbooks! I'm blessed to have such a caring person in the publishing world.

God—my Creator. He gave me a cancer cross to carry— but He also helps me carry that cross. Through God all things are possible! I'm very thankful that God's Hands helped my hands write this book.

Table of Contents

Introduction

The old saying goes, "When life hands you lemons, make lemonade." It's really good advice to suggest making the best of a bad situation, and it's always been one of my strongest beliefs. I even added to that familiar motto when I first started creating healthy recipes.

My version of this slogan became, "When life gave me lemons, I not only made lemonade, I wrote the recipe down, and I sold it!"

Nearly fifteen years ago, I turned a life-threatening health problem—losing more than one hundred pounds—into a successful career as a cookbook author and motivational speaker. I took a bunch of negatives—all those extra pounds, and the medical concerns that accompanied them, such as high blood pressure, gout, and arthritis pain—and created a new life shaped by a positive attitude and a determination to change.

It just made sense to me back then, in 1991, to strengthen

my own motivation to help myself get healthy by sharing with others what I was learning about how to live healthier. Now, with more than thirty cookbooks, a monthly newsletter, a public television cooking series, and other books on how to live a healthier lifestyle, I can see the evidence that my efforts to "make lemonade" from those old lemons have paid off in so many ways.

But it's never been just about my own success. In getting to share what I've learned with others, I feel that I've fulfilled one of the most important missions in my life on this earth. I've always felt blessed to have been given the opportunity to touch so many lives.

By the time I turned fifty-seven, I thought I had a pretty good idea how the rest of my life would unfold—that I'd be working less and enjoying it more, that I'd be spending time with my children and grandchildren, that I'd keep growing my gardens and writing my newsletter and learning more about the tricks my computer can do.

But destiny and the Lord had plans for me that I never expected. I woke up one morning and discovered that the world as I knew it had changed forever. The journey that followed that discovery was the spark that created *this* book—one I hope will be a gift to my readers, old and new, as I share what I've learned while traveling down this unexpected road.

A friend once said to me, "Life is what happens to you while you're making other plans." How true that is! But life is also what you do with what happens to you, how you meet the difficulties, confront the challenges, and overcome the obstacles that life places in your path.

In this book, I'll be sharing my recipes for living through a crisis that took me almost to the edge and back. (I've also "tucked in" a few recipes of the usual kind: my Lucky Seven Lemon Recipes!) This story doesn't have an ending yet, and I hope it won't have one for many years to come. But I think it's a tale worth telling, and it's one that I hope will touch you, encourage you, and even help heal what ails you.

You see, I'm convinced that I never would have made this journey as well as I have without you. Thank you for being part of my support team. Now I hope I can persuade you to let me be part of yours.

How My Life Changed in a Moment with a Diagnosis of Cancer

I expect that you may already know quite a bit about me, if you own any of my Healthy Exchanges cookbooks or if you've seen me on QVC or on your public television station over the past dozen years. Maybe you've read a few issues of my food newsletter or heard me speak at the Iowa State Fair, or at an RVers' convention, or for hospital diabetic and cardiac support groups all over America.

But for those of you who don't know much about me, let me introduce myself as I do when I speak to groups these days. I am JoAnna Lund of DeWitt, Iowa. I'm a wife, a mother, and a grandmother. I'm also a businesswoman and a cookbook author who's famous for her healthy recipes—especially pie! I'm an avid gardener, a pretty good seamstress, and a voracious reader.

But I'm also a Stage IV inflammatory breast cancer survivor. And while all of these different hats that I wear have taught me plenty, right now I want to share what I've learned from my experiences with this life-altering disease. They truly have helped me turn one of life's sourest lemons—a diagnosis of cancer—into lemon meringue pie.

Not every important life event has a clear beginning, but this one does. About four years ago, I went to bed one evening, here in DeWitt, in my own bed at Timber Ridge Farm after an ordinary busy day of recipe-testing, answering e-mail, and working in my garden.

But the next morning when I awoke, I discovered that my left breast had turned bright red and become as hard as a rock. The skin of that breast resembled an orange peel, all dimpled, and there was a strange, odorous discharge coming from the nipple.

You can probably imagine my first reaction. I'm sure my blood pressure and pulse escalated, as I experienced a mix of confusion and fear. It felt almost as if something had taken over my body, like in the movie *The Invasion of the Body Snatchers*. Suddenly there was this part of me that I had paid little attention to and didn't seem to belong!

Then the part of me that always responds well in a crisis snapped into action. "Calm down," I told myself. "Calm down. It can't be anything serious, because nothing serious would happen this fast." That made sense to me, and I felt myself start to breathe more normally.

Something was clearly wrong with my breast, but what? Then I remembered, way back when I was a young mother and nursing my babies, I'd developed a case of mastitis. My breast had been red and swollen and hard because of an infection of the milk ducts. Now, even though I was years into menopause, could I somehow have developed it again? The more I thought about it, the more I decided that I was right. The way my breast looked and felt really mimicked mastitis.

So by the time I showered and had my clothes on, I had already given my condition a name. I called it "menopause mastitis." Now all I needed was to get confirmation of this from a medical professional. My family doctor had recently retired and moved away, so I decided to go to a woman's clinic not far from my small town and have my "condition" checked out.

Later that morning, I called the woman's health clinic in Davenport, Iowa, and made an appointment. Because I had convinced myself by now that it wasn't anything serious, I didn't tell them it was an emergency. I just took the next available appointment for a new patient, which was about six weeks away. Then, as luck would have it, when it got close to the time for my appointment, I had to cancel it to handle an emergency in our business. So I called the clinic and asked for the very next one instead.

An Infection, or Something Worse?

During all this time, nothing had changed. I had no pain. I wasn't tired. I didn't feel sick. All I had was this funny-looking breast. I was still convinced it was nothing more than an infection.

I had always heard and believed that you were supposed to check your breasts for lumps, and if there were no lumps, you didn't have to worry. I do have to admit that I hadn't gotten yearly mammograms, but my doctor hadn't pushed for them. He had just thoroughly examined me, including my breasts, during periodic physicals and nothing had ever shown up. There was no history of cancer in my family, and my doctor had never found a thing.

About eight weeks after that first morning I noticed the reddened, hardened breast, I finally saw the doctor. She did the usual parts of my exam, and then she started doing a check of my breasts. She manipulated them, examining both carefully. Then she asked me how long my left breast had been that way and I told her, "Oh, about a couple of months." I added that I thought it was an infection.

She told me that she, too, would have thought that it was an infection and probably would have given me antibiotics if I hadn't told her how long I'd had the condition. She said, "If it *was* an infection, it would have cleared up by now on its own. Otherwise, it would have become so painful that you would have been crying for help."

Then she paused, and for the first time I heard the words: "It may be cancer."

I have since learned that many general practitioners react just as I did, thinking, it looks like an infection, so it must be an infection. Most women with inflammatory breast cancer lose as much time as I did, maybe even more, by the time the doctor realizes that the antibiotics aren't doing what they should.

In Shock

After I heard those words *"It may be cancer,"* I was in a kind of shock. My sense of confusion only deepened when she added, "What surgeon do you want to go to? I want you to get a biopsy on this right away." Well, I didn't know what to say. I didn't know any surgeons who dealt in cancer. It seemed so unlikely that I might have cancer. Me, out of everyone else in the family?

I never smoked.

I never drank.

I never did drugs.

I was never sexually promiscuous.

I was never a sun worshipper.

I was always in bed by nine and up by five. (More than two hundred years earlier, Ben Franklin had promised that anyone who did that would be "healthy, wealthy, and wise"!)

For the past twelve years, I had committed myself to living

a healthy lifestyle, eating healthy food, getting moderate exercise, making lifestyle changes—and always keeping a positive attitude.

So when the doctor asked me which surgeon I would like to see, I told her, "I don't know anyone. You just send me to whomever you think is the very best and who believes in God."

Lucky for me, the surgeon she called happened to have an opening that afternoon. I called my sister Jeannie and asked her if I could come over to her house to wait until my appointment. Of course she said yes, but wanted to know what it was for.

"The doctor wants me to be checked out to make sure I don't have breast cancer."

Then I called my husband, Cliff, and told him I wouldn't be coming right home. I must have sounded like I felt, because by the time I got to Jeannie's, my other sister, Mary, was already there. Fifteen minutes later, Cliff arrived; he must have driven down to Davenport really fast.

So all four of us went to the surgeon. On the way, my sisters kept insisting that it couldn't be cancer, that there was no history of cancer in our family. But I think I already knew what I was going to hear from the surgeon.

It was fast. He took one look at me, and the very first words out of his mouth were: *"I'm almost certain this is inflammatory breast cancer."*

Well I'd heard of cancer, I'd heard of breast cancer, but I had never heard anyone talk about something called inflammatory breast cancer. But before I could ask him all the questions that were bubbling up in my brain, he added, "Before we can properly diagnose this, we'll need to do a biopsy, and I also want you to get a mammogram."

I have since learned that even if I'd gone for a mammogram a week before this reared its ugly head, in all likelihood I would have been sent home with a clean bill of health. That's the scary part. Once it exploded like a volcano, so to speak, it was calcified, and the mammogram picked up the calcification. (In medicine as in life, timing is everything, I guess.) The doctor who had looked at the films asked me, "Now, it's just your left breast they're concerned about?" And in response to my questioning look, she answered, "Well, there's a lump in your right breast as well." It was a lump that wasn't caught in the physical exam—the kind that is so small, it is almost invisible. It's the kind that mammograms are intended to catch.

So—in a matter of hours, I went from thinking, *I just have an infection,* to finding out, I *probably have cancer in both breasts.*

I headed back to the surgeon, and he did biopsies on both breasts. He broke three needles doing my left breast, and for him that confirmed his diagnosis of inflammatory breast cancer, because he told me it had only happened to him a few times in the past, and each time, it was IBC. Moments later, he shared that the lump on the right side was so small, he felt it could be treated easily with a lumpectomy and there would be no problems whatsoever. Then he said, "Oh, but the left side . . ."

I began to cry, and asked, "What do you mean?" He said, "When you go home, you need to start doing research on the Internet on inflammatory breast cancer, because that's what this is." Then he said, "It's going to have a huge impact on your life." I asked, "Why?" to which he replied, "Well, you have less than a fifty-fifty chance of living five years."

Okay if I scream now?

Screaming is not my style. But to actually hear someone say that you might die so soon is downright scary.

The surgeon then asked, "Who do you want for your oncologist?" But since I wasn't on a first-name basis with any cancer doctors, I said, "You just send me to the very best doctor you know of in the Quad Cities—someone who will allow me to ask as many questions as I need and who believes mightily in the power of God." Without much hesitation, he responded, "I have just the man for you."

Then he added, "We have a meeting every week among the surgeons and oncologists in this area, and we always discuss new and interesting cases. You will be the topic of conversation this week, even before you see him."

And so, knowing the biopsies would be ready in a few days, he made an appointment for me with the oncologist for the next week, on Christmas Eve day.

The "Verdict"

The oncologist told me that yes, I definitely had cancer in both breasts. It's a diagnosis that would terrify any woman, and I was no exception. I didn't feel sick, and I didn't look sick, but it turned out that I was very sick indeed.

He suggested that I have several rounds of chemotherapy to shrink the cancer, then a double mastectomy (removal of both breasts), probably followed by more chemo and then radiation. He added, "But we won't do anything until after the first of the year, because right now the hospitals and the clinics are half staffed."

I'd already made plans to fly down to San Antonio to spend the holiday season with my daughter, Becky, and her family, and he thought it would be the best medicine for me anyway.

Shortly after the Christmas holidays, I had all my baseline tests—tissue, bone, and blood—as well as X-rays and a lot of other tests too numerous to mention. Three days later, on January 5, I had my second appointment with the oncologist, and that's when I heard even more frightening news: There was cancer in every lymph node under my left arm. It had spread to my entire chest wall, it was in the outside skin of my left breast, and it had traveled to more than a dozen places in my bones.

My oncologist answered every question I asked and told me what I needed to understand. He then suggested, considering how aggressive my cancer was, that I not have the double mastectomy, unless I insisted. It would be locking the barn door after the horse had already bolted away. Instead, he said, we would start on a very, very intensive chemotherapy protocol—doctor-speak for a course of treatment with a particular drug.

He also suggested that I go buy a wig *now*, while I had the energy and the hair to which to match it. So on my way home,

I stopped at a wig shop and almost as if it were waiting for me, I saw *my wig* on a mannequin on the counter. It was my hair on a good hair day—the exact same color and style.

So I bought it, thinking that probably within two to three weeks I would be wearing it. Well, I was wrong, and the doctor was wrong. Even though I was on adriamyecin—a chemo drug notoriously known for causing hair to fall out in a matter of weeks—I never lost my hair, and five chemo protocols later, I've still never put that wig on. In all likelihood, I probably never will. But I'm saving it as a souvenir.

Keeping my hair was the first little miracle I experienced after my diagnosis, but I hoped it wouldn't be the last. (At the time, I had no idea how many ups and downs I would experience as I fought for my life and tried to keep my sanity—and my sense of humor!)

This journey has been a series of miracles—physically, emotionally, and spiritually. And I hope that my thoughts, reflections, and prayers, as well as those of many others who have inspired me, will help you cope, thrive, and prevail over whatever life crisis you're facing now. Together—yes, together—we can do it!

"Grandma's" Lemonade

My life changed in an instant when I learned I had cancer, but some good things never change—like the sweet and tart flavor of old-fashioned lemonade made easy for the twenty-first century!

❀ Serves 8 (1 cup)

> 1 tub Crystal Light sugar-free lemonade mix
> 8 cups water
> ¼ to ½ of a lemon, unpeeled and unseeded

Prepare sugar-free lemonade according to package directions. Slice ¼ to ½ of a lemon, including skin and seeds, into chunks. Pour 2 cups of prepared lemonade into a blender; add lemon chunks and blend on HIGH for 30 to 45 seconds. Pour into the pitcher of lemonade mixture and mix well. Serve over ice and enjoy!

HINT: You can also use ¼ to ⅓ of an orange for Lemon-Orangeade, or ⅛ to ¼ of a lime for Lemon-Limeade.

Each serving equals:

HE: 1 Optional Calorie

1 Calorie • 0 gm Fat • 0 gm Protein • 0 gm Carbohydrate • less than 1 mg Sodium • 0 gm Fiber

DIABETIC EXCHANGES: Free Food

(from: *The Healthy Exchanges Cookbook*)

Recipes for Healing

Finish each day and be done with it. You have done what you could. Some blunders and absurdities no doubt crept in; forget them as soon as you can. Tomorrow is a new day; begin it well and serenely and with too high a spirit to be cumbered with your old nonsense.

—Ralph Waldo Emerson

Healing happens at so many levels, beginning at the microscopic. You make peace with an old enemy, and your body feels a tiny rush of positive energy. That "rush" may knock out a few cancer cells or encourage the pieces of a shattered bone to start mending together. I'd like to think so, but I don't really know if this happens.

What I do know is that it's up to each of us to help heal ourselves when faced with a crisis, to create a spiritual climate of wellness inside ourselves. So when I began organizing my thoughts and "recipes" for this book, I felt that what I'm calling "healing" would be the place to start. For me, this is the place where I'd like to help you prepare your mind and heart for the journey ahead. It's up to you to choose how you are going to handle the many emotions of this challenging time, and to consider the big questions that become so important in times of crises.

When I look for healing, I start with the Lord, but I also listen to my own heart and the precious words of others on this path called life.

❖

Choose how you will react to your health crisis, and you'll feel better already. Isn't it amazing?

We can't always control what's happening to our bodies. For me, that includes the effects of the cancer itself, or the results I get from the chemo; for others, it means the outcome from surgery or from radiation or another treatment.

But we *can* control how we react to what's happening.

How did this happen? How did *I* end up so sick, with a really serious form of cancer? Well, of course, all kinds of people get sick. I guess the question most of us can't help asking is, "Why me?"

Well, when I did ask, "Why me?" I answered my own question: "Why *not* me?" If someone in my immediate family was going to get cancer, probably it was better that it happen to me. I certainly wouldn't want it to affect my daughter or daughters-in-law, who are caring for their young families. Nope, all things considered, I would rather cancer be "served on my plate" than to any other family member.

I *can* cope with cancer, I discovered through trial and error.

See, that's what you do. That's what "healing" is. You figure out a way to live with what you've got to live with, or else you give up—and you don't get to live your life. You consider your choices, you make your pick, and you live with it—emphasis on the "live!"

I discovered that I felt this way almost from the beginning. I liked my oncologist immediately, because he "heard" me when I said I wanted to know my options. (He still makes recommendations when they're indicated, but the ultimate choices are mine.)

I was originally supposed to have a double mastectomy soon after I was diagnosed, and while I found the prospect scary, I was certainly willing to do it to save my life. But after all the initial tests were completed, my oncologist told me that instead of surgery, he wanted to start me on an aggressive program of weekly chemotherapy instead of the usual monthly treatments. I got *less* of it *more* often, instead of *more* of it *less* often. (It turns out he was ahead of the curve in his advice to me. Now, this approach is pretty standard.) He felt that I would "get with the program" and do what I needed to get through this.

Did I fully know what that would mean at the time? I don't think so. But I sent a silent message to my body, agreeing to partner with it in this healing process—and somehow, my words got through.

From the beginning, I've had chemo almost every Friday. For someone who was in the habit of working six days a week, I have to admit it was something of a shock to have to take every Friday off to devote to my treatment.

But I've learned that while chemo rules my Fridays, it doesn't have to rule my life.

Now, instead of working so hard, I look at my Fridays as *my day*. First I get my chemo treatment, and then I spend the rest of the afternoon doing whatever I choose to do on that particular day—depending on how I feel, of course.

Sometimes, I head for the nursery, picking out new flowers to plant in my gardens. Sometimes, I visit local thrift shops in search of special cookbooks that I need to complete a set I'm collecting. Sometimes, I enjoy going shopping for myself or for one of my family members. Other times, I choose just to spend time with my sisters and just talk.

The bottom line is, I've chosen not to dread Fridays and the infusion of chemo because I know it's helping me to live longer, maybe long enough to see my grandchildren grow to adulthood. By combining my treatment with pleasurable activities, I've moved my Friday focus from treating my cancer to enjoying how this change in my schedule has also changed my life for the better. I can face my chemo more positively because I know the rest of the day is mine to enjoy in whatever way I choose.

As I write this, spring is in the air. It's only a matter of weeks before I can again be outside digging in my gardens. As Duke, our precious golden retriever, and I walk around our property, breathing in the fresh, earthy scents, the harsh winter months are not only forgotten, they are forgiven. We stroll from the fruit orchard to the vegetable gardens, inhaling the wonderful aroma of nature awakening from a long winter. We wander from the ponds across the firm, damp ground to amble past the flower gardens.

Occasionally, my husband, Cliff, joins us on our daily walks, but usually it's just Duke and me. As we roam around the farm, I often use the time it takes to cover our ten acres to think. This morning, for instance, as I watched with pleasure the first budding of so many of the plants and shrubs I'd planted last year, I began to think about forgiveness, and how great it would be if people could be more tolerant and forgiving, just as plants and animals seem to be.

Have you ever noticed that even when we neglect our weed-pulling duties, flowers and plants push their way up through the earth anyway? It's as if they know how much we need their beauty and passion to grow to reignite our own desire to dig into the loamy dirt and connect with nature. Even when there hasn't been enough rain, they draw sustenance from whatever they can to keep going. Even when the sun has hidden behind clouds for days in a row, they don't give up, they don't surrender to despair—because they know that rain and sun will return again.

I feel that it's the same with animals, who offer their affection even when we have been inattentive or too caught up in our own lives to seek them out. They seem to understand that whether or not we express our need for them, it's always there. They don't judge us by our actions but by a kind of belief and expectation that we will answer kindness with kindness, if only just given the chance.

But are people that understanding and forgiving of each other? Do we give each other the benefit of the doubt, endless second chances to make something right?

※

Alma Gaul, our local paper's Erma Bombeck, wrote a wonderful article on the subject of forgiveness for the Sunday *Quad City Times* a while back. I asked if I could share her words with you, and she agreed.

FORGIVING IS THE INGREDIENT OF A HAPPY LIFE

Did you read the story last week about what makes humans happy?

According to psychologists, the happiest people are those who surround themselves with family and friends, do not care about keeping up with the Joneses, lose themselves in daily activities and, most important, forgive easily.

Oh. And I was doing so well on this list . . .

One of the trickiest things about forgiveness is the need to forgive people who haven't asked.

That is, sometimes people really tick us off—are unreasonable or unfeeling—and they, darn them, don't see it that way! They see no reason at all to ask forgiveness because they see nothing unreasonable or unfeeling about what they did or said.

Well! This is tough. But to harbor a grudge against these people just eats away at ourselves, causing a diminishment in *our* quality of life and lets them off scot-free! So, for our own health, we need to find a way to forgive these people.

It isn't easy, because forgiveness isn't just a mental exercise. It's difficult to will into being something we don't feel. There are those who say that "forgiveness is a gift so profound that it can only come from God."

We have to work at it, or ask for help, or both, depending on our outlook.

The other tricky thing about forgiveness is that it is ongoing.

That is, we don't necessarily do it just once, but over and over again every time we see the person who offended us.

One thing that helps is to force ourselves not to dwell on wrongs. The more we dwell, the harder resolution can become. Once we've thought a thing through and made our decision on how to deal with it, we need to go on. Think about something else. It takes a tremendous amount of energy to carry a grudge.

It also helps to remember what someone once told me—never attribute to malice that which can be explained by stupidity.

That is, don't take offense at every annoying thing that is said or done because often no offense is intended. The other person is simply oblivious, so we should be, too. Otherwise we're investing effort in something that doesn't deserve it. Dumb.

And, finally we must forgive ourselves. We all do wrong and give offense at times. Once we've made an effort to make amends, then we need to let it go.

❖

It's good to remember that we *choose* how to respond to the acts and words of others, that the power is within us to decide how we will feel about what others say and do. This is such an important realization, especially for someone coping with a serious illness like cancer.

In order to live without the dead weight of anger and disappointment, of bitterness and loneliness, we need to practice forgiveness in all kinds of ways.

We need to forgive the comments of an acquaintance or even a friend who may think she is being sympathetic or helpful, but whose words cause pain: the neighbor who can't seem to resist sharing stories of family members who suffered painful treatments for the same disease; the well-meaning colleague who asks if you've started putting your affairs in order; the insensitive workmate who inquires if you've selected a grave site or will opt for cremation.

It's harder, but just as important, to find a way to forgive someone who suggests that something you may have done caused your illness or made it worse. How do you react to a health-care worker who thoughtlessly notes that your obesity may have made you more likely to develop breast cancer, for instance, since some research has indicated that higher levels of estrogen in overweight women may contribute to the emergence of the disease? What can you say in response to someone's comments that she spied you at a local fast-food outlet with your grandkids and haven't you heard about the carcinogens in those grilled burgers?

(None of these have actually happened to me, but I've read such posts on cancer support group websites, so I know that they do happen!)

Is it right to respond with anger, to send the person away feeling ashamed or embarrassed?

I don't think so.

It takes precious energy to generate a nasty reaction, energy I can't spare for the purpose. It takes time and a willingness to let bad feelings build inside me, and I just don't have the time or the desire to feel that bad about something so insignificant.

It's easier to forgive.

It's easier to say to myself, That person must still be so full of anguish over the painful experiences of her relative that she has to keep talking about it. I can do her a kindness of listening without judging her—and without getting angry that she is sharing such negativity with me when I need just the opposite.

It's better to forgive.

It's better to say to myself, This person who asked if I'm putting my affairs in order may simply be trying to be practical. He may have learned firsthand that people who are unable to think about or plan what they want at the end of their lives can create emotional chaos for their families. He may have been thinking that it's better for people with serious illnesses to choose a health-care proxy, make a will, even imagine their own funerals, while they are still feeling strong enough to ensure that their wishes are carried out.

Remember the old quotation from Shakespeare? "To err is human, to forgive, divine."

It's "divine" to forgive.

Divine means something close to God, and perhaps nothing could be more appropriate than to forgive someone whose words or actions hurt us. As the Bible quotes Christ, "Father, forgive them, for they know not what they do." Doesn't that seem like an appropriate response to negative, hurtful, tactless, and insensitive acts or remarks?

A health-care worker who casually "blames" a patient for her own disease may not see herself as cruel, but such comments don't do anyone any good, so why make them? While it might seem reasonable to say that someone who smoked caused their own lung cancer, the fact is that many people who develop this type of cancer never smoked at all.

You could get angry, you could lash out, you could even decide to banish such a thoughtful or misinformed individual from your life.

Or—you could forgive them for not knowing (or perhaps even caring) what they say. That way, you have the power to decide what happens to you, instead of surrendering that power to anyone else.

❖

Okay, so it's good to forgive others. But we also need to find a way to forgive ourselves.

What other people say often echo things that we've already thought. And even if we've managed to quiet those thoughts for a while, it's easy to ignore them but it's not so simple, if you hear the same notions from a friend or colleague, or read it on the Internet.

Many people coping with cancer or other serious illnesses face this problem of self-doubt. I certainly did. From the very earliest days of my diagnosis and treatment, I had to come to terms with the question of whether my cancer would have been caught sooner or been less serious if I'd had regular mammograms. Or, if I'd insisted on an immediate appointment with a doctor instead of accepting one that was some weeks later.

Would I have developed inflammatory breast cancer if I had been a size six instead of a generously proportioned woman whose hips have always been a size larger than the rest of her?

Did anything I unknowingly did in my life, from where I lived to what I ate to the kind of tests my doctors ordered, cause my cancer to grow silently inside me?

Most of us ask these kinds of questions because we want to place blame somewhere, even if it's on ourselves. And all too often it becomes easier to blame ourselves than something or someone else.

But rarely can even the most skilled researchers pinpoint exactly what caused an individual's cancer or what a patient might have done differently to prevent that illness from developing.

I decided very early on that I had to set these concerns aside and that I must forgive myself for anything I might have done to influence or affect my cancer diagnosis. My strong, practical nature tells me that there is just no point in stewing about it now. What's done is done, and now all that matters is how I handle the challenge of getting better.

So that's what I did. I forgave myself (even if it turned out that nothing I could have done would have changed the outcome) and I moved on to my real focus: working with my medical team to do the best I can . . . *the best I can,* to fight my disease and continue to live my life.

Forgiveness is power.

Forgiveness is a gift you give yourself and others.

Forgiveness is positive energy that can overpower the negativity of anger, disappointment, regret, and guilt.

Each morning, as you thank God for the gift of a new day, add forgiveness to your gratitude. Decide to forgive those who have hurt you—whether it was intentional or accidental, a sin of commission or omission. You will feel the glow of goodness, not only in your heart but in your body, as you get on with living!

❖

Live every day as if you expected to live forever but might die tomorrow.

—Author Unknown

I don't get to many Broadway shows, but occasionally I hear songs from them played on the radio. At least, that's where I think I first heard one of the most moving songs from the award-winning musical *Rent*. The song, "Seasons of Love" begins by counting "Five hundred twenty-five thousand six hundred minutes," then goes on to ask how you measure the moments and the meaning of a year in a person's life.

How many sunsets, and how many midnights? How much laughter, and how many tears? How many cups of coffee, and how many truths learned? And do we remember to celebrate, with joy and with recognition those precious minutes, all 525,600 of them, in each and every year of life?

I've heard people say that when they were young, a year seemed to last forever. Kids keep asking, When am I going to be big enough to do this or that? Then somewhere around your late twenties or early thirties, time seems to speed up . . . and all of a sudden you find you want it to slow down!

By the time you reach midlife and beyond, and you start to realize that you may have more of life behind you than in front of you, time becomes more precious than it ever seemed before. Still, even knowing that your allotted years, months, weeks, days, and minutes are slipping away, do you feel that you're not making the most of your God-given time?

I think parents may be more aware of this passage of time, because they see their children growing up before their eyes. One moment you're teaching a little boy to walk; the next, you're running beside him as he learns to ride a bike; and soon, you're cheering him as he runs the length of a football field.

It seems impossible when the child you gave birth to is now nursing a little girl of her own, and it feels so strange the first time someone calls you Grandma. You sort of look around to see if your mother-in-law is there, and suddenly you realize that you're the grandma now.

I'm not the only one thinking about how precious time is now. One of my newsletter readers e-mailed me a beautiful cyber-essay. Its original source is unknown, but the sentiments it expresses touched me as much as I hope they will speak to you.

TIME . . .

Imagine—there is a bank that credits your account each morning with $86,400. It carries over no balance from day to day. Every evening it deletes whatever part of the balance you failed to use during the day. What would you do? Draw out ALL OF IT, of course!

Each of us has such a bank. Its name is TIME. Every morning, it credits you with 86,400 seconds. Every night it writes off, as lost, whatever of this you failed to invest to good purpose. It carries over no balance. It allows no overdraft. Each day it opens a new account for you. Each night it burns the remains of the day. If you fail to use the day's deposits, the loss is yours. There is no going back. There is no drawing against the "tomorrow." You must live in the present on today's deposits. Invest it so as to get from it the utmost in health, happiness, and success! The clock is running. Make the most of today.

To realize the value of ONE YEAR, ask a student who failed a grade. To realize the value of ONE MONTH, ask a mother who gave birth to a premature baby. To realize the value of ONE WEEK, ask the editor of a weekly newspaper. To realize the value of ONE HOUR, ask the lovers who are waiting to meet. To realize the value of ONE MINUTE, ask a person who missed the train. To realize the value of ONE SECOND, ask a person who just avoided an accident. To realize the value of ONE MILLISECOND, ask the person who won a silver medal in the Olympics.

Treasure every moment that you have! And treasure it more because you shared it with someone special, special enough to spend your time. Remember that time waits for no one. Yesterday is history. Tomorrow is a mystery. Today is a gift. That's why it's called the present!

One of my favorite verses from the Bible, and which I think about more now than ever before is from Ecclesiastes:

> *To everything there is a season,*
> *a time for every purpose under the heaven.*
> *A time to be born and a time to die;*

a time to plant and a time to pluck up that which is planted;

a time to kill and a time to heal;

a time to break down and a time to build up;

a time to weep and a time to laugh;

a time to mourn and a time to dance;

*a time to cast away stones and a time to gather stones
    together;*

a time to embrace and a time to refrain from embracing;

a time to get, and a time to lose;

a time to keep and a time to cast away;

a time to rend and a time to sew;

a time to keep silent and a time to speak;

a time to love and a time to hate;

a time of war and a time of peace.

Reading over this beautiful text, I can't help making connections to so many of the lines. When I say aloud, "A time to be born," I think of the astonishing miracle of birth, how I felt when my own three children arrived in this world, from God's hands to mine, and how I have felt each time I've been blessed with a grandchild who carries a little piece of me in his or her body and soul. If one definition of "miracle" is that it's something that defies human understanding, perhaps the miracle of birth is one of those, for even as we understand the biology of how a child is made and born, it still seems an act greater than anything we know how to do on this earth.

The line continues then, "A time to die," and I recall the passage of so many people that I have loved and been loved by——my parents, my grandparents, my wonderful aunts and uncles, my father-in-law, and so many friends. I carry their memories inside me for all of my life, and so while they may have died, they will never truly be gone from me. As I grow older, and as I recognize that the years in front of me are fewer than those I have already lived, this Bible verse speaks to me of a kind of acceptance of God's great plan for all of us.

I always smile when I hear, "A time to plant, and a time to pluck up that which is planted." You can't live your life in Iowa and not feel the changing of the seasons as farmers experience them, even if you are not a farmer yourself. You become aware of the changing of the seasons as you drive along the highways lined with cornfields in their many stages of growth. As the stalks grow, as the corn ripens, as the harvest nears, so, too, the year moves on, a day at a time, each day required to bring all those magnificent ears to their most golden and beautiful color.

It's harder to make peace with the next words, "A time to kill, and a time to heal," and yet we accept them as we accept the blessings of freedom. My children served in the Gulf War, and while I deeply sympathize with every mother and father whose child now stands on the same kind of front lines, I know that sometimes battles must be fought before a nation can be healed and a world brought to true peace. As it was in the beginning, so it has been generation after generation.

"A time to break down, and a time to build up" says to me that our landscape is ever changing, and yet it never loses its recollections of what has gone before. When we first broke ground for our home here at Timber Ridge Farm, I thought about the history of this land, imagining Native Americans and pioneers hunting deer and tending vegetable gardens centuries before. At times like that, time seems so fluid, and only the land remains a solid memory.

"A time to weep and a time to laugh"—oh, how those words resonate for me now, for this experience of disease and treatment has overflowed with tears at times and yet never managed to squelch my ability to laugh at silly things or a child's sweet words! Sometimes I have found myself laughing and crying all at once. It's not unlike a scene from the movie *Steel Magnolias,* when a grieving Sally Field cannot suppress a burst of laughter on the day of her daughter's funeral. She tells her friends that she's so angry, she wants to hit something, and Olympia Dukakis pushes Shirley MacLaine forward and suggests that Sally "hit Ouiser," suggesting that Ouiser sacrifice herself for the greater good. It's such an outrageous comment that all the women present (except poor Shirley M.) begin to laugh at the situation. Sally Field's character is embarrassed and even a bit horrified at her ability to grin, but her hairdresser buddy played by Dolly Parton tells her that "laughter through tears is my favorite emotion!"

Ecclesiastes shows us again that two warring emotions are aspects of the same thing, in "A time to mourn and a time to dance." To me, a perfect example of this is how a parent feels when a son leaves for college or a daughter gets married. You can't help mourning the loss of childhood and those special joys of parenthood that can't really last, and you must find it in your heart to celebrate, joyfully, the new life your son or daughter is about to embark on, with a dance. I wept and smiled when Becky first danced with her husband at her wedding. (I also, of course, wept when Cliff gave her away—and smiled all at the same time!)

It's so much the same with the following lines—you must be willing to let your children go even as your heart pleads to hold on tight; you may gather to yourself beautiful things that give you pleasure, but also understand that giving them away also brings remarkable satisfaction; you should choose your words wisely and learn that sometimes it is better not to say something than to express what you're feeling or thinking.

Ultimately, life is all about time and how we use it. The sooner we learn how precious it is, the better use we make of it. As I reflect on the many aspects of my life, I've come to realize that time is really my most important and valuable commodity! Maybe it's because I'm now forced to think of my own mortality in what I call AD (After Diagnosis) Time in ways I never did in BC (Before Cancer) Time.

Doing the Really Important Things, First

The other day, I received a call asking me to schedule an appointment for a radio interview on a particular day. In BC days, I might have moved heaven and earth to make myself available, but now I'm comfortable saying, "Sorry, I have plans that day. Can we make it another time?"

What were my plans for that date? A "just the girls" journey into our nearest big city for lunch and shopping. My sisters, Mary and Jeannie, and I now make it a priority to "do lunch" often or drive into Chicago just to visit and shop. We're all still busy—but we now make the time to be together. We always go during the week, which surprises friends and colleagues who "knew me when."

In the past I would not have dreamed of taking a workday off for *pleasure,* but I do it now. I won't do it every day, but I am sure going to do it when I want to. I'll enjoy the day for all it's worth, being with my sisters, eating someplace new, finding things for my table settings that I wouldn't have found otherwise. We shop cheap, and that's the fun of it, finding bargains and bringing them home to the farm. It's just plain fun. I'm doing something I love—spending time with my sisters, creating memories.

What better way to spend precious time? And who knows, perhaps what better way to heal the emotional bruises that facing and fighting my cancer has caused?

Even Cliff and I have changed the way we schedule our daily lives. We're committed to spending quality time together that's *not* about business! These days, when Cliff's home from the road, we both stop work much earlier than we used to back in BC Time, even if it's just to spend our early evenings talking or watching TV. Nothing exciting, but definitely enjoyable—and time well spent, which keeps us close.

Finally, the time I spend working on my gardens, either planning new projects or tending to existing ones, is private time that I cherish. I feel like I'm connecting with God as I go about my gardening tasks. So while I'm planting and raking in my Garden of Hope and Healing, I'm really praying as well. This special garden is an emotional work in progress; as I plant decorative grasses by the pond or find the perfect spot for a contemplative bench, I'm really expressing gratitude to our Father Almighty for the time He is granting me to devote to my gardens.

As I continue on the road to recovery, I plan to share this garden with the residents of our local nursing homes, so they, too, can connect with God in this Living Prayer of Thankfulness.

Now, I decide how to spend my time—no one else does.

I've been "healed" of needing the approval of others before feeling free to enjoy each hour of my day in my chosen way. What better time is there than now to make the break from living only for others—and live instead for yourself?

The time I spend on Healthy Exchanges endeavors is time I consider well spent. I still love creating my "common folk" healthy recipes and sharing my common-sense approach to healthy living as much today as when I first began! When I get busy on this project or that, hours seem like mere minutes. Sometimes I look up to see that I've been working without a break for quite a long time. That's another way I know that I've chosen a good way to spend my precious time, because I become unaware of its passing!

Time spent with my family is even more valuable now than it ever was before. I look forward to my daily phone conversations with my daughter, Becky. I dearly love learning what her children, Spencer and Ellie, are doing today that they weren't doing yesterday. I enjoy hearing what's new with her husband, John. And I like catching up on Becky's new decorating projects. These may seem like mundane subjects to other people, but they're oh-so-special to me!

Now, there was a time when I didn't talk to Becky every day, a time when we were both so busy and involved with our own lives that we didn't always make the time. *Now we do.* Now we understand that our times together are some of the best times we have all week!

It's the same situation when my son James and his wife Pam and their precious sons drop by the farm for an unexpected visit. Whatever else I'm doing can wait. And when the boys can stay overnight, it's pure heaven, even on those days when I'm tired from my chemo treatments. Zach, Josh, Aaron, and Abram bring me more pleasure than all the gold in Fort Knox ever could!

They say that when you look back at your life, you won't regret that you didn't spend more time at work—but you will regret not spending more time with your family. That's why, when my son Tom and his wife, Angie, and their little girls, Cheyanne and Camryn, come for a stay, I carve out as much time as possible to spend with them. I treasure every moment spent applauding while Cheyanne sings and dances. And the little girls and I love our "private time," whether we're sharing secrets or when I'm painting their fingernails a pretty pink— just like Grandma's!

Not every grandma is lucky enough to spend so much time with her grandchildren, but I'm grateful for every occasion. I'm making memories with these wonderful kids, and after I'm gone, I hope those memories of me will stay with them always!

Take a moment today to think about how you might make your own special memories. I believe it's a healing choice to shift the emphasis in our lives, no matter our ages or even our illnesses, from the work we produce to the time spent with people who need us. It's not only about family time, either. I know people whose families are far away, but who devote some time each week to tutoring a child in reading or working in a food pantry. You can even reach out without leaving your home—I've read of wonderful programs where volunteers call homebound neighbors and make powerful, healing connections with those who would otherwise languish isolated and alone.

Imagine—you have a gift more special than you may have imagined: the power to heal others even as you heal yourself!

A New Attitude

The following story, one of many that has found its way to me via the internet, appealed to me because it took me into the kitchen—my favorite room in the house—to teach me a valuable lesson about how we see ourselves.

CARROT, EGG, OR COFFEE?

A young woman went to her mother and told her about her life and how things were so hard for her. She did not know how she was going to make it and wanted to give up. She was tired of fighting and struggling. It seemed as one problem was solved, a new one arose.

Her mother took her to the kitchen. She filled three pots with water. In the first, she placed carrots; in the second, she placed eggs; and in the last, she placed ground coffee beans. She let them sit and boil without saying a word.

In about twenty minutes she turned off the burners. She fished the carrots out and placed them in a bowl. She pulled the eggs out and placed them in a bowl. Then she ladled the coffee out and placed it in a bowl. Turning to her daughter, she asked, "Tell me, what do you see?"

"Carrots, eggs, and coffee," she replied.

She brought her daughter closer and asked her to feel the carrots. She did and noted that they got soft. She then asked her to take an egg and break it.

After pulling off the shell, she observed the hard-boiled egg.

Finally, her mother asked her to sip the coffee. The daughter smiled as she tasted its rich aroma. The daughter then asked, "What's the point, Mother?"

Her mother explained that each of these objects had faced the same adversity—boiling water—but each reacted differently.

The carrot went in strong, hard, and unrelenting. However after being subjected to the boiling water, it softened and became weak. The egg had been fragile. Its thin outer shell had protected its liquid interior. But, after sitting through the boiling water, its inside became hardened.

The ground coffee beans were unique, however. After they were in the boiling water they had changed the water.

"Which are you?" she asked her daughter. "When adversity knocks on your door, how do you respond? Are you a carrot, an egg, or a coffee bean?"

Think of this: *Which am I?*

Am I the carrot that seems strong but with pain and adversity, do I wilt and become soft and lose my strength?

Am I the egg that starts with a malleable heart, but changes with the heat? Did I have a fluid spirit, but after a death, a breakup, a financial hardship, or some other trial, have I become hardened and stiff? Does my shell look the same, but on the inside am I bitter and tough with a stiff spirit and a hardened heart?

Or am I like the coffee bean? The bean actually changes the hot water, the very circumstance that brings the pain. When the water gets hot, it releases the fragrance and flavor. If you are like the bean, when things are at their worst, you get better and change the situation around you.

When the hours are the darkest and trials are their greatest do you elevate to another level?

How do you handle Adversity? Are you a Carrot, an Egg, or a Coffee Bean?

Don't tell GOD how big your storm is. Tell the storm how big your GOD is!

For me, the diagnosis of cancer was an incredible wake-up call. I was finally faced with the fact that I may not have many more days or years, so I want to spend them wisely. I discovered that I have more compassion, and I understand better how easily time may be frittered away because of circumstances beyond my control. I find that choosing what to do becomes easier, not harder, because I have a new clarity: I'm just not going to waste precious days and weeks and months doing what I don't want.

All the same, I'm more frugal with my time; ironically, I'm likely to be less concerned or upset over minor disappointments or delays. It's just not worth the energy anymore. Isn't that a relief?

I believe that my attitude may well be part of the reason that my cancer has responded so well to the treatments I've received. I went into chemo as a person who'd made a career of "living healthy in the real world." I had long given up on ever being "Hollywood skinny" and instead appreciated being real-world healthy, as I saw it. I'd made peace with myself, and with the hips that always ran a size larger than the rest of me. I was never going to be glamorous, but I'd promised myself to enjoy life to the fullest!

Is it reasonable to think that my lifestyle before I discovered I had cancer—the healthy food, the moderate exercise, and a truly positive attitude—was one of the primary reasons that I was able to reverse the tide and respond to my treatment? Sure, why not? I also wasn't taking any medicine when I started my chemo, so my body was able to respond right away instead of having to swim through a lot of other chemicals in order to zero in on the cancer.

At the same time, I knew that getting better would take a lot of energy I'd previously devoted to other activities. So I made a deal with my body: I get to remain busy and active, but I know my limitations, and I don't try to exceed them—not too often, anyway.

I need to be in this for the long term, not for quick fixes. Now that time is more precious, it's important to see the distant reward, not just the immediate ones. My goal, I decided, was to see my youngest grandchild graduate from high school. Whatever your goal may be, you'll want to examine your choices each day to make sure that what you're doing will help you achieve it.

✲

I'm not looking for miracle cures or unproven hype. I just want to do whatever I can to help my doctor help me help *myself*. And I know that optimism—doing my best to stay positive—helps.

That's not to say that I never have a moment of sadness or disappointment. Of course I do—I'm human, and I'm dealing with a disease that can be terrifying at times. But when I find myself edging toward negativity or misery, I *choose* to stop and regroup. Instead of succumbing to the darkness of cancer, I keep looking for those glimpses of light, those "candles in the darkness." By making a special effort to rediscover what's good in my life, I can use that positive energy to help my body heal.

Illness or crises of any kind bring out all kinds of emotions, from fear to anger to frustration, and all those little things you think won't affect you emotionally turn out to be the ones that do. I get weepy over the silliest things, things that never used to affect me so much. That's just part of what I've come to call my "new normal." And part of that is making a daily effort to think and be positive.

Discovering the Purpose in Our Lives

Did you know that your attitude can be *positively* contagious? It's true. When you keep putting one foot in front of the other, when you face any test with a cheerful demeanor and an optimistic spirit, all those around you will likely find it easier to lift their own hearts.

My oncologist told me about a patient he treated whose depressed state just made it harder for her to fight against the cancer. Then, in a matter of days, he observed a genuine transformation, a complete turnaround. He asked what produced the change in her outlook, and she replied that she had been in the same chemo room with me three or four times. She added, "If JoAnna can keep a positive attitude with what she's facing, then I guess I can, too."

Does that justify why I'm going through all this? Or why anyone goes through any trial? I started thinking that maybe the purpose behind my own cancer journey is to help someone else get through it, maybe more than a few "someones." If I was going to willingly accept a cross to bear, this is *not* the one I would choose. But it was chosen for me, so I'm not going to ask why. I'm just going to do the best I can . . . *the best I can,* and someday it may be revealed to me—if not on earth then, I hope, in heaven.

I've been an outspoken person all my life, the type of person who doesn't keep anything private, and so what better-suited unofficial spokesperson for this rare but deadly form of breast cancer could there be? If I can help other people cope with their disease, and maybe help save their lives, that's just fine with me.

When I heard the words *"You have cancer,"* I coped by finding out everything I could about how to fight for my life. I wanted to know all the possible weapons I could use to beat back this opponent. But at the same time I "stockpiled ammunition" to fight this potentially deadly disease, I prayed to God about what I was feeling.

I said, "God, I choose to fight my cancer because I feel there's so much I still want and need to accomplish in my life. But I also choose to accept this trial in whatever way You want me to."

As I prayed, I got a real sense of what God's answer was.

I felt that He wanted me to fight.

I felt that He had plans for me that required me to keep going, to stay here on earth to do His work—and mine.

So I found myself asking a *different* kind of "Why me?"

Why am I still here, practically in remission after being diagnosed in Stage IV? I know that in just the few years since I was diagnosed, there have been a lot of good people who found out they had cancer—people who are no longer here.

I know it's not because I'm a better person or because I prayed harder. I just think it's because God has other plans for me. So that's how I'm going to proceed.

Life is God's novel. Let Him write it.
　　　　　　　　—Isaac Bashevis Singer

Lemon Fruit Salad

When you're feeling stressed-out by your treatment and too tired to spend much time in the kitchen, this old-fashioned fruity combo is just the thing to lift your spirits and perk you up!

❈ Serves 8 (⅔ cup)

1 (4-serving) package JELL-O sugar-free instant vanilla pudding

1 (4-serving) package JELL-O sugar-free lemon gelatin

⅔ cup Carnation Nonfat Dry Milk Powder

1 (8-ounce) can crushed pineapple, packed in fruit juice, undrained

¾ cup Diet Mountain Dew

½ cup Cool Whip Free

1 (8-ounce) can fruit cocktail, packed in fruit juice, drained

1 (11-ounce) can mandarin oranges, rinsed and drained

1 cup (1 medium) diced banana

In a large bowl, combine dry pudding mix, dry gelatin, and dry milk powder. Add undrained pineapple and Diet Mountain Dew. Mix well using a wire whisk. Blend in Cool Whip Free. Add fruit cocktail, mandarin oranges, and banana. Mix gently to combine. Cover and refrigerate for at least 15 minutes. Gently stir again just before serving.

HINT: To prevent banana from turning brown, mix with 1 teaspoon lemon juice or sprinkle with Fruit Fresh.

Each serving equals:

HE: 1 Fruit, ¼ Fat-Free Milk, ¼ Slider, 6 Optional Calories

108 Calories • 0 gm Fat • 3 gm Protein • 24 gm Carbohydrate • 231 mg Sodium • 80 mg Calcium • 1 gm Fiber

DIABETIC EXCHANGES: 1 Fruit, ½ Starch/Carbohydrate

(from: *Cooking Healthy with the Kids in Mind*)

Recipes for Support

A true friend reaches for your hand and touches your heart.
—Author Unknown

It's 4 A.M. I'm wide awake and alone with my thoughts, and my fears. This feeling isn't unique to cancer patients, but I sometimes think that we feel more alone than other people in crisis because we know we're in a fight for our lives—and that's a scary place to be.

I was famously independent for much of my life. Before I met my second husband, I raised three children on my own, worked full-time, and went to college. I got used to the feeling of being in charge of my days and nights. I don't know if I completely bought into the idea of "if you want something done right, do it yourself," but I may have acted as if I did on many occasions.

Not anymore.

I've learned that I don't get extra credit from the Lord or anyone else for struggling through tough times all alone. Relying on friends and family is a healthy choice, and even finding solace from unseen "angels" through the Internet can make the difference between sleepless nights and sweet dreams.

The ingredients of support are many and varied. You may have to take the first step yourself and ask for what you need, but you'll discover an abundance of help out there just waiting to be tapped!

Balthasar Gracian, a Spanish philosopher, wrote these wise and beautiful words on friendship more than four hundred years ago:

> "Have friends. It is a second life. Remember, we have either to live with friends or with enemies, therefore try daily to make a friend. . . . Be not too fragile in bumping against the world, and least so with your friends; for some crack with the greatest of ease, showing that they are made of poor stuff. Such trifles bruise them that real hurt is not necessary. So search out those who promise to last . . ."

He goes on to say that,

> "Knowing how to keep friends is more than knowing how to make them. True friendship doubles the good and divides the bad. It is the only defense against misfortune, and the very balm of the spirit."

Isn't it remarkable that a person born centuries before I was can speak to my heart as if he were in the room with me as I write this? I'm learning that time and distance seem to know no boundaries when it comes to friendship. And sometimes a stranger will reach out across the miles to offer healing words and inspirational stories that give us the courage to go on.

Quiet Angels

May there be peace within you today. May you trust God that you are exactly where you are meant to be. I believe that friends are quiet angels who lift us to our feet when our wings have trouble remembering how to fly.

It's more than a little amazing that on the same day, another e-mail included the quotation: "Friends are kisses blown to us by angels."

※

Remember when you were just a baby (well, okay, you may not actually remember, but stay with me on this . . .) and you were learning how to walk? Your little legs first struggled to stand on their own, but they wobbled, and so in order to move from where you were to Mommy's arms or to reach a favorite teddy bear, you looked around for support. Maybe you grabbed a table leg, and then a chair. Maybe you propelled yourself along while holding on to the wall. You did whatever it took to get where you wanted to go—and it didn't matter at all that you couldn't do it without a little help.

Getting through tough times is a lot like that.

You can't survive if you can't get from here to there, but in order to do it, you need to look around for whatever kind of support will help you accomplish your goal. It's never more true than when you're responding to a crisis, particularly one that involves your own health.

For most of us, the closest source of support is family. My sisters, my husband, and my grown children are, and have always been, the "rock" upon which I've built my life. But for many people whose parents may no longer be alive or whose siblings may live far away, friends have taken on the role of family. Most of the single women and men I've spoken with over the years have confirmed this for me. Whether your dearest friends go back to elementary school years or have sustained you since you began working together in recent years, they are sure to be the rock upon which you will build your support system to help you sail through the rough waters ahead.

Friendship isn't a big thing—it's a million little things.
—Author Unknown

Do you take even your closest friends a little bit for granted? Too many of us do. We expect them to be there when we pick up the phone, and we sometimes go for days, weeks, or even months without checking in—even as we tell ourselves that the bonds that hold us together are strong enough to survive.

In the introduction to her book *The Love of Friends,* Barbara Alpert, my friend and collaborator, wrote:

"They are the family we choose to surround us, sisters bound by love instead of blood. They know when we are lonely and appear without being called. When we feel lost, they provide a living map to what comes next; when we doubt everything about ourselves, they remind us who we are.

"Our women friends are the richest treasure we possess, and the importance of friendship in women's lives cannot be overemphasized. These precious, powerful relationships sustain us when everything else seems in flux; if we're lucky, our friendships may endure for decades and across thousands of miles."

She goes on to say that,

"True friendship is not only a gift but a responsibility, a commitment," and she adds that in some ways, "A friendship is exactly like a marriage, with a vow, spoken or simply understood, to love and honor each other in soul and spirit, to stick by one another through thick and thin. In a very real sense, true friends commit to those they love for richer and for poorer, in sickness and in health. No license is signed, no ceremony witnessed, but the bonds of friendship are so often stronger than those that join a man and woman together."

Her words ring so true to me, as I think of many of the friendships I've had since childhood. They certainly outlasted my first marriage, and some of my oldest friendships are stronger now than they were even a decade ago.

When I close my eyes, I can see us as we were then and as we are now.

We've survived raising teenagers and finding gray hairs.

We've lost (and gained back, and lost again) hundreds of pounds.

We've supported each other whether the crisis was a broken-down car or a broken-down marriage.

We've laughed and cried together so many times we've lost count—and we've been there for one another through the best of times and some of the worst, too.

The friends who keep our secrets and encourage our dreams are so important, we must make time to cherish them and make sure they know how much we love and depend on them.

When I picked up Barbara's book recently, it fell open to a short quotation from renowned television journalist Linda Ellerbee. It turns out that she and I have more than one thing in common: "To say old friendships are best is trite, and like so much that is trite, true. Two years ago, I was diagnosed with breast cancer. I learned I would lose both breasts. Carol and Judy flew to New York to be with me, to make me laugh, to let me cry. Other, newer friends were there for me during that time, too. But only Carol and Judy had, as they pointed out, known me before I grew breasts to begin with."

One of the benefits of growing up in a small community is that the school classes are much smaller. Back in 1962, my graduating class from Lost Nation, Iowa, was tiny, fewer than thirty kids. Everyone in town knew everyone else, which could sometimes feel claustrophobic but mostly made us feel cared for and safe.

Not long after I was diagnosed with breast cancer, I was both touched and astonished when Dawn and Sherry, two of my classmates (since first grade!) and also two of my oldest friends, decided to launch a very special "get well" campaign on my behalf. They contacted every single person in our graduating class and asked them all to send me cards on the very same day. Well, before I knew it, I started receiving this giant "card shower" from my classmates from all over the United States. Hearing from them, knowing they were praying and hoping the best for me—it was just incredible. Some of them I hadn't heard from for years before this!

It gave me such an emotional boost to know that I was remembered so fondly all these years later. It just proved to me that while we may not see each other as often as we used to, when push comes to shove, they are still folks I can count on for encouragement and support.

Don't be shy about sharing good and bad news with old friends, through alumni newsletters or church bulletins. The people who cared about you years ago probably still do, and they may consider it a blessing to be "invited" back into your life at a difficult time.

�֎

A hug is an amazing thing—it's just the perfect way to show the love we're feeling but can't find the words to say. It's funny how a little hug makes everyone feel so good. In every place and language, it's always understood. So here's a BIG one just for you! (The following poem was sent to me, unattributed, some time ago and I am taking the liberty—with thanks to the anonymous author—of sharing it here.)

HUGS

There's something in a simple hug that always warms the heart.
It welcomes us back home and makes it easier to part.
A hug's a way to share the joy and sad times we go through.
Or just a way for friends to say they like you cause you're you.
Hugs are meant for anyone for whom we really care.
From your grandma to your neighbor, or a cuddly teddy bear.

✖

Some friends come to us later in our lives. They arrive by chance, or as I prefer to think of it, serendipity. Our paths simply cross because of something we've both decided to do at the same time. But our friendships can't be explained away just because of convenient geography. There had to have been something in each of us that needed something in the other, a part of us that found a kindred spirit in a stranger who quickly became a friend.

When I discovered that I had cancer, I also found that some of these friends were a splendid source of comfort during times when I felt a bit worried about my reactions to my chemo or a little discouraged that my energy wasn't as high as I wanted it to be. Just when I needed it, there would be an e-mail or a card from far away, sent by the "veterans" of our Healthy Exchanges cruises with whom I'd grown so close during our sojourns at sea. Over the past several years, they've come to visit us and helped us relive some of those eventful and exciting days afloat. Others who live farther away regularly call to visit over the phone. It's lovely to chat about other destinations we might head for someday, making some glorious new memories to add to our scrapbooks and fill our hearts!

Don't be afraid to reach out now, while you're right in the middle of chemotherapy or other treatment. There is just no better time to reconnect with people who have shared the bits and pieces of your life so far. They can help energize you and give you a real sense of hope for the future—the reason you're trying so hard to live through this crisis!

⁂

More treasured support has come from other friends as well. The women I work with at Healthy Exchanges are my employees, it's true, but we've been together for a very long time and the ties between us go pretty deep.

When I first brought everyone together to tell them about

my cancer diagnosis (because I wanted them to hear first from me before they heard it from anyone else) Jean told me that she had been thinking about retiring, but said that now there was no way she was going to leave. She's continued to work part-time, and her loyalty means a lot.

Shirley, who's been typing my recipes since the very beginning, has been a friend for longer than we both can measure! She just does anything and everything on my projects to make it easier for me, and she will rearrange her own busy life to help me meet my deadlines.

Gina, who's my assistant, has also taken on a lot during this time. She makes sure that when she's scheduling my appearances, I don't get overextended. If I agree to do one speaking engagement in the evening, then she won't plan any more for the rest of the day.

Rita, my chief recipe tester, works around my chemo and my good days. She is there for me without complaining that one week she has to work *these* days, and next week maybe it will be other days instead. I depend on her more now than I ever did before, and she has come through for me again and again.

Does it surprise you that a boss was open to help from her staff? It shouldn't. I needed them to help me do what was still very important to all of us—keep my business running while I was treated for my cancer. By making them a part of the team, I benefited more than I can say—but they've also told me that they felt good doing something to sustain the company that is their livelihood.

✸

Have you ever heard the expression "Strangers are just friends we haven't met yet"? When I decided to share the facts about my cancer in my Healthy Exchanges newsletter, I got e-mails and letters from just about everywhere! People sent their best wishes and told me that they'd put me on their prayer lists. (I think I am being prayed for in just about every church denomination and synagogne in the country!) Hearing that meant a lot to me, because I believe the collective power of prayer is mighty.

Very soon after my diagnosis, I also decided to tell the food editor of the *Quad City Times,* who's done so many wonderful stories about me, and I also contacted the host of a TV program in Davenport. From the very beginning, both have supported anything and everything I'd ever done, so I wanted to let them learn of my cancer diagnosis directly from me. Both of them asked if I would mind going public with my story so that maybe we could educate and encourage others.

I was a bit hesitant but I agreed, and within a month, I'd been written up in the paper and also talked about my illness on TV. As word spread, thousands upon thousands of people sent me cards. Each one was like a boost of energy, or an embrace from a friend! (I'd always been someone who sent cards for special occasions, but now that I know how much they meant to me, I send a card practically at the drop of a hat!)

It's been a humbling experience in some ways, to know with every envelope I open that people I've met only through my books, newsletter, and cooking demonstrations have taken the time to write to me and put me in their prayers. What an act of friendship that is, especially when we may never have come face to face. There hasn't been a day since I first shared the news of my illness that someone hasn't cheered me up by finding a few precious moments to drop me a line!

Does it seem excessive to describe these communications as evidence of friendship? I don't think so. A friendship can begin in a moment, as a spark can give birth to fire, and friendship can and will grow into a warming blaze with just a little effort. Recognizing friendship is another gift that must be cultivated, so we don't accidentally miss the signs that someone is reaching out to us.

❋

I know it's hard enough to find quality time in our busy lives to share with our families, but if you believe, as I now do, that friends are the relatives we choose for ourselves, then it's vital to s-q-u-e-e-z-e in some "girlfriend time" somehow and somewhere. So maybe your kitchen floor won't be clean enough to eat off, but who wants to eat off the floor when you have such a lovely kitchen table—and another table in the dining room?

Two of my dearest friends, women I first got to know back when I was a young farm wife, recently decided that we needed to spend more time together. Even though our lives have taken different paths, and we're all very busy in our own endeavors, we got out our calendars and figured out when we could meet. For years, we hadn't spent near as much time together as we did when our kids were little, but now that our kids are having kids, we wanted to change all that. So we decided to get together for lunch every few months to do nothing but talk, talk, talk! That may not sound like very often, but our wonderfully long lunches are perfect for catching up and sharing the latest photos of our grandchildren.

> *Love seems the swiftest but it is the slowest of all growths. No man or woman really knows what perfect love is until they have been married a quarter of a century.*
> —Mark Twain

For some of us, an important part of our support system sleeps (and maybe snores!) in the bed next to us. Of course the marriage vows promise "in sickness and in health," but that doesn't mean that every spouse is able to deliver on that pledge.

My husband, Cliff, and I have just recently celebrated our silver wedding anniversary. It is a second marriage for both of us. I was a thirty-five-year-old working mother with three young children. Cliff was a long-distance truck driver who seemed so much more mature than his actual age of twenty-eight. When we first met two years earlier, we were both going through the trauma and misery of a divorce, and we found that we could help each other through that ordeal.

When Cliff became my husband, he also willingly became the instant father of three. And father he was, and is to this day, in every sense of the word. In fact, a few years ago, my daughter, Becky, jokingly told me, "Mom, if you ever get divorced, we kids get custody of Cliff!"

Our relationship has survived business crises and personal ones; we've watched our children grow into remarkable adults and we've become grandparents of eight healthy and beautiful grandchildren; we've traveled all around this country in our mobile home as I did my book tours, and we've seen each other at our best and worst.

Or at least I thought we had, until I received my diagnosis of Stage IV inflammatory breast cancer. I'm a strong woman, but I will tell you this flat out, it's a comfort to have a man to lean on when trouble comes your way. And Cliff's the best kind of "leaning-on" man. He doesn't get overly emotional, but he also doesn't run when I get that way—and sometimes I do.

He made me believe, on that difficult day, that we were in this together, and that together we would make it. I think he knew how much I needed to hear that from him.

He's always been there for me, no matter the challenge I faced. When I began creating my Healthy Exchanges recipes, he promised to eat just about anything I put in front of him (well, except dishes featuring broccoli or shrimp!) as long as it tasted good. He's been supportive of my work from the beginning, when I borrowed $2,000 from the bank to print copies of my first, self-published cookbook, and he's done just about everything, from driving the motor home up mountain passes and along bumpy roads to selling cookbooks at State Fair appearances, from repairing the printing press to getting my newsletter to the post office, all the while acting as my chief taste-tester.

Our relationship has changed over the years, but our willingness to be flexible and open to changes in how we live and work has sustained us, and it's helped us get through some of the toughest times. We've changed our plans as life has changed us, but we've learned that change doesn't have to be forever—it just has to be right for the time you make it.

※

Now, some changes aren't a choice but occur without warning. You won't know before they happen how you and your loved one's will handle them when they do. And there's probably no greater test of a marriage than finding out that one of you has cancer.

Cliff passed this one with flying colors.

Who knew? True, when I married him, I'd already seen how he dealt with the pain of his own divorce. He'd helped me through my own, too, and over the years has been a source of strength. But the true test of a man—well, let's just say that when you vow "in sickness and in health," you're promising a lot more than you know!

The first week I went for my chemo, Cliff went with me, and the nurse explained in detail what side effects might occur, but we still didn't know what to expect. I got chemo on a Friday afternoon and was still okay most of Saturday. We were having an open house on Sunday for my mother-in-law's eightieth birthday. We had been planning it for months, and I wasn't going to cancel it, *not* because of my cancer diagnosis and *not* for my first chemo treatment.

I felt a little queasy Saturday night, so I went to bed early. At midnight I woke up—and I just started going off like Old Faithful. I can't even begin to describe it. Without one cross word or a single complaint, Cliff (who would never clean up after kids, pets, or anything), cleaned me up, cleaned the bed up, cleaned the rug up, and two hours later did it all over again. (And, I might add, without so much as a grimace on his face.)

The next day, I was exhausted, so I just stayed in my bedroom with the door closed. As many of our more than two hundred guests heard for the first time about my diagnosis, I lay in bed imagining they were thinking that I was on my deathbed. Well, I wasn't, and I'm not. But I'm thankful to Cliff and to my wonderful family members who kept the party going and did a fabulous job.

Since then, there have been more than a few rough times, where Cliff has come through without a whimper. Sometimes I get these sudden, unexpected fevers when my blood counts are too low, and I develop infections. Now we know better what to do, but the first two or three times, in the middle of the night when my temperature was 102 degrees and I was freezing, Cliff would bundle me into the car and rush me to the emergency room, because that's what the doctor had said to do. No matter what time it was, no matter the weather or his own exhaustion, he never once complained.

Another time, I experienced really severe leg cramps because one of the chemos didn't agree with me. I started having these intense muscle spasms that hurt me so much. Cliff got up, again in the middle of the night, when I was in such awful pain, and he massaged my legs, putting hot, wet cloths on them and helping me walk.

These are the times that test a marriage, that test a relationship. Some pass and some don't. Well, Cliff did better than pass. He aced it!

※

I'm lucky to have Cliff. But I know that not everyone facing a crisis can rely on a spouse to come through. For some, it may be the surprise of a sister, long-estranged, who leaves her home and family for weeks to care for a loved one. I've heard from others who were astounded when a relative who wasn't even that close showed up and stayed as long as she was needed. And there are still others who don't have a single family member to comfort and confide in—but who are touched by a neighbor's offer to drive them to doctor's appointments and keep them nourished when the effort of cooking a meal is too much.

But this kind of support is a two-way street. You need to reach out and accept help when it's offered instead of hiding away or letting fear, pride, or shame keep you isolated and alone. And sometimes you need to ask for what you may desperately require—and if you're someone who's always taken satisfaction in handling your own problems, that can be very hard.

I think it may be one of God's lessons for us—that we are born into this world as part of a community, and even if we have lost touch with that reality, He wants us to relearn it, now in this time of anguish and grief. Giving others the opportunity to share God's love with you is a gift for both the giver and the receiver.

※

Sometimes it's the little things that mean so much, that make an astonishing difference in your daily life, when you're coping with cancer or a serious health threat. But you don't have to wait for someone to read your mind. Share your concerns and people will come through for you. You'll discover that many caring friends and family members want to do *something*—they just don't know what, until you tell them!

I'm organized in many ways, but more than occasionally my life gets chaotic—and something I need to do falls by the wayside. Cliff decided that one way he could help was by making sure I took my medication without fail. He fills my seven-day pill container each weekend and makes sure that my prescriptions are filled when they run low.

But not every act of kindness is as critical as making sure I take my medicine. Years ago, Cliff had made it clear that if we were going to have cats, I would be the one who took care of them. But when I started chemo, the nurses told me not to tend to their litter box because of potential contamination. Cliff agreed that we didn't want to get rid of the cats, so he took over that task. It's been more than three years now, but he's never complained once.

Cliff's also begun doing things that I enjoy that he might not have done in the past. He gladly digs the holes for my plants now, and in BC Time he didn't. He liked lawn mowing, so that was his contribution to "our gardening projects." Now, though, I think he enjoys working in the yard with me as I do with him.

I really like to listen to uplifting radio programs, like Dr. Dobson's *Focus on the Family*, where they solve everyday problems with everyday practical advice. And I also love to watch the Gaither Homecoming Southern Gospel concerts every Sunday morning on TV. They're on pretty early, but Cliff gets up and watches with me because he knows how much they mean to me. (He doesn't really care much for talk shows on the radio, and he prefers country-western-type music to gospel, so I appreciate his willingness to listen to what I like. He started doing it out of his feelings for me, but now he enjoys it, too!)

And even my daughter-in-law Pam, who's been a real God-send for me, comes over every Wednesday night to help me clean my house. Pam and the boys come for supper, and then after she takes the boys to their Royal Rangers church group, she comes back to the house and cleans while I rest until it's time to go get the kids.

Little things mean a lot more than you can ever imagine.

※

I know that it's not always easy accepting help, especially when you feel you can't do anything to "return the favor." But there are ways you can show your appreciation by giving yourself, your attention, and your time.

On most Sunday afternoons, Cliff loves to watch NASCAR on television. Until recently, I used to leave the room and do something else—work on the computer, sew, or watch a different show on another TV. But now I sit there with him. I bet I don't know any more about auto racing than I did for the first twenty-plus years of our marriage, but I know that *he* enjoys it more because I'm there with him. It's a little thing that represents a real change in attitude for me. And because it means a lot to Cliff, I now enjoy my time sitting there with him.

Team Spirit

Remember that old inspirational slogan: TEAM—Together Everyone Achieves More? Well, it's not just a string of empty words used by business executives to motivate their sales forces during a slow season. It's true in just about every area of our lives. While there are some creative jobs one usually does alone (writing, painting, composing music, inventing recipes), in almost everything else we do, we benefit enormously by the assistance and input of others.

Are you one of those people who views asking for support as a sign of weakness or insecurity? Have you stood proudly and said, "Yes, I did it all by myself"? It's good to "own" your accomplishments, of course, but I've discovered firsthand how valuable and vital support can be to help me do what I want to do—and since I was diagnosed with breast cancer, to "get me through the night"!

If you've ever been a member of Weight Watchers or TOPS (Take Off Pounds Sensibly), if you go to AA meetings or have attended Parents Without Partners, you already know that the support of a group can be the difference between success and failure, between achieving a goal of better health or succumbing to bad habits and unhealthy actions.

From my earliest days online I'd thought that Internet support groups would become a powerful lifeline for so many people, and they have exceeded even my early expectations. If you're a new mother up at 4 A.M. with a colicky baby, you're not alone anymore with your worries. Log on, and you're likely to find kindred spirits all over the Web who can answer your questions and put your worst fears to rest.

The Internet, in its unique way, has turned a world of billions of people into a giant small town, where at any time you can get answers to all kinds of questions (from "How many teeth does a corn snake have?" for a child's report to "Has anyone experienced numb fingers and toes from taking this medicine?"). Whether you seek out an actual support group or simply search through the America Online member directory for someone who might be able to help, you may be astonished to discover just how many people are eager to share their knowledge and provide comfort!

Our son Tommy insisted way back in 1995 that we start a Healthy Exchanges website (www.healthyexchanges.com). This was years before many businesses had much of a presence on the Web, but he felt we should do it—so we did. He said to me that in just a few years, running a business without a website would be like running a business without a phone.

I could see that having a website would be a good way to share my weight-loss success story and my healthy living program. But Tommy figured we could also use it to promote and sell my cookbooks, and even alert readers when Cliff and I would be coming to their towns on a book tour. He also envisioned a time when my readers would want to be able to contact me and each other. And how right he was!

What the rest of us didn't understand at the time was how powerful the Web could, and would, become. From the time we launched our message boards and chat room, we created a place for people from all over the country (and even the world) to listen in and learn from each other.

Some who first met on the boards went on to develop e-mail friendships; others discovered they were practically neighbors or lived only miles apart, close enough to arrange face-to-face meetings!

I learned so much by stopping by to read the posts and listen in to the chats. I got terrific feedback about my recipes and eating plan, and I experienced real satisfaction in "hearing" how real people had incorporated my suggestions and transformed their lives.

But I was also very moved by observing how virtual strangers gave so much of themselves in order to help each other. Folks who were following a weight loss program but not attending regular meetings found some needed (and welcoming) group support; people struggling to make necessary changes in their lives got powerful encouragement from people they'd never met.

Over the months and years, I've found myself deeply touched by the different stories shared on the site: inspiring tales of weight lost and health regained, discouragement and disappointments the writers felt free to share only with their online pals; sorrowful discussions of how it felt to cope with the loss of a spouse, the challenges of a disability, or even a serious, life-threatening disease.

It was my first experience with this unusual, now common, type of support group—but I don't think I ever imagined that I would need to seek out the same kind of emotional and informational sustenance for myself just a few short years later!

As soon as I received my diagnosis of inflammatory breast cancer, I spent hours searching for information on a variety of websites, many of which are listed in the Resources section in the back of this book. But a lot of what I needed to know wasn't available on the sites that provided the facts about tests, treatments, chemo, and the newest drug protocols. I had a million questions, and while my doctors were incredibly open and willing to answer just about any question I asked, they couldn't answer them all.

I needed to talk to other people who also had my disease.

I wanted help sifting through all the statistics, the pages and pages of diagrams and single-spaced warnings about each and every drug prescribed for women in my situation.

I ached to know about what I could do—and not do—during my treatment.

I wondered how others were coping with everything from the side effects of their medication to the aftereffects of regular chemotherapy treatments.

So I went looking for an interactive website where I could "lurk" for a while until I got my bearings, then begin to ask questions—and share my myriad concerns about this unexpected new wrinkle in my life!

I found a number of different options and decided to join a few: an inflammatory breast cancer support group (www.ibc-support.org) and one called BC Mets (www.bcmets.org), for those whose breast cancer has metastasized (spread to other parts of the body). (I also joined a HER2 support group for those who are HER2 protein-positive—more on that in the Resources section.) Finding those other women (and a very few men) out there in cyberspace definitely saved my sanity—and it probably helped save my life, too.

While I visited some general breast cancer sites, I chose an inflammatory breast cancer online support group because this is a relatively rare form of cancer, and our concerns are somewhat different from those of many women with breast cancer. It was a tremendous comfort to discover, for instance, that many of the women had had no advance warning before IBC erupted in their bodies. By sharing the details of our symptoms and our treatments, the members of the group have helped each other immeasurably. We've learned what to expect after different types of chemo, and we've shared warnings about what we shouldn't do while on particular medications.

We've also been there for women who are trying to decide

which of several treatment options to choose. Recently, one woman asked our group for advice when she was told her cancer had spread so fast, it probably wouldn't help her much to have her breasts removed in a double mastectomy. But she was more than a little uncomfortable walking around with, as she described it, "breasts filled with cancer."

The group suggested that she contact me because I experienced the very same situation. I told her, as I always do with anyone who asks me for specific advice, that healthy living solutions are just like panty hose—one size definitely does not fit all. I told her that she had to do what she thought was best for her, and that it helps to have real trust in your oncologist and your medical team.

I told her that I didn't feel the least bit uncomfortable walking around with cancer in my breasts. Why? Because I've decided to look at this as a chronic condition. I compared it to the situation of someone walking around with a heart that's damaged. But everyone is different, I reminded her, and she is entitled to have the feelings she has.

It turned out that the drugs I took for my inflammatory breast cancer reduced the tumor of regular breast cancer in my other breast. Another person might not have the same experience. It's a tough decision. Some doctors—but certainly not all—may recommend *not* having cancerous breasts removed because of the difficulties of the recovery period and the potential risks of postoperative infection. Again, it depends on the individual, and it depends on the medical advice that is offered.

I believe that my doctors and I made the right decision for me, and so that was what I suggested this woman do: talk to her doctors, get a second or third opinion if she felt it would help, and then put it in God's hands. In the end, that's all we can really do.

I know that I've tried to share with others as much encouragement and positive attitude as I can. I like to say, you do what you need to do to go on and you do what you want to do because this is your life. I don't dwell on the fact that there's cancer in my breasts. Instead, I rejoice in all I can do each and every day *in spite of it*.

❖

Online support groups give new life to that old motto, "Two [or more] heads are better than one." Even if you spend hours a day looking for information on the Web and from outside sources, you won't find *everything*. There's just so much information, you simply can't! But when you all put your heads together and share the good news, the helpful tips, or even just regular words of encouragement and "This, too, shall pass," you make it better for everyone involved!

I e-mailed the happy news of my first remission to my four online support groups—my Healthy Exchanges Group, my Inflammatory Breast Cancer group, my BC Mets group, and my CookbooksEtCetera group (a spirited band of avid cookbook collectors from far and near). I got wonderful replies from members of every single group—messages sent to me personally and others sent to the group as a whole. It took me several weeks to answer all of the personal messages, but I kept at it! (I always feel that if somebody cares enough to write me a message, I need to acknowledge it and write back.)

The cookbook-collecting group went one step further. Mo, who leads the group, invited everyone to a "Virtual Party," a cybercelebration at her house by the ocean! Here's some of what she wrote:

"The southern California sun is shining at 70 degrees today, slight ocean breeze, so all of you in the northern states where old man winter is overstaying his welcome can come get a little SoCal sunshine. . . . Bring your special dish to the brick patio. . . . Watch out for the piñatas hanging from the avocado tree. . . ." Then she went on: "This is a happy occasion we are celebrating with JoAnna, who has been fighting for her very life the last two years. What a fighter she is! I think God was listening to our prayers for her and decided she really did have too much to do down here on Earth before she could go home."

She ended her invitation, "What are you bringing? Where are you coming from? Why are you attending? How can YOU add to this wondrous party for our friend?"

Then the replies started coming, as dozens of members shared great little stories about how they were going to get to the party and what tasty dishes they were planning to bring. Each one touched my heart and brought a smile to my face.

One woman said she'd paddle over from Hawaii in her canoe

and bring a ukulele boy along so we'd have music at our party. Another said she was going to rent a private jet and have a friend fly her out. And oh, the food! We were going to feast on every possible delicacy, from stone crab claws (Florida) and pork ribs and bar-b-que sauce (Texas) to peaches and pavlova (Australia) and forty-eight bottles of wine (the Netherlands). One woman said she'd prepare three hundred homemade spring rolls; another promised to set up a "monster crawfish boil" and also bring huge pots of seafood gumbo from New Orleans. Still others offered Maine lobsters, chocolate mousse cake, Red Thai beef, cookie dough truffles—the list went on and on!

This cyberfest went on for more than a week in real time, as we planned a weeklong celebration at Mo's. We shared all the things we had to celebrate and talked about the days in life we'll never forget: the day we start school, the day we're married, the day we had our first child, and the day we had our first grandchild.

Now, one of the great things about a cyberparty is that it takes place in the heart and the mind. This was one celebration where no one *but no one* was worried about counting calories—they were bringing their very best "cyberfood." That's why everyone's imaginations felt free to stretch creatively! I told them I'd be bringing Lemon Meringue Pie, of course, and Grandma's Lemonade as my contribution.

In the end, Mo and I decided to gather up all the correspondence and created a little memory book just for our members, all those who joined in the celebration. We included all their e-mails describing how they'd get to the party and who and what they were bringing, along with recipes for the dishes that they wanted to serve. I sent one to everyone who was part of this memorable event! It was so uplifting to be treated this way, to have my friends from far and near want to celebrate this very important event with me. I will always remember it, and I think they will, too.

It's the little things—things that don't cost anyone any money, take just a little time, that are remembered long after anything else. When diamonds are lost and money spent, memories of such kindnesses will last forever.

So how do you find this kind of energizing and comforting on-line support? It's simple—simpler than you may imagine.

And don't worry, because no one will make you participate until you're ready. You can read the posts on the website of your choice, you can "lurk" and "listen" and draw strength from what you find there.

Truly, you don't *ever* have to talk live with anyone if you don't want to. You don't have to respond to a single posting if you don't feel like it. If you're not comfortable becoming part of an e-mail round-robin (a sort of group e-mail setup), you don't have to join one.

On the other hand, I hope you *will* join in, because sharing your thoughts and your fears not only helps you, it helps *you* help *others*. You'll discover that no matter how isolated you may feel or how alone with your thoughts and your concerns you think you are, there are other people out there who may share exactly your worries and situation.

If your first experience to a site leaves you unsatisfied, don't give up. Try again a few days later, or find another site and group that may fit you better. And if you don't have a computer at your disposal yet, consider signing up for regular time at your public library. Your Internet visiting is your own business, even when you're away from home.

Now what about finding support in person? Is it just too old hat? Not at all. Just as many people are willing to drive an hour to attend a Weight Watchers meeting, others are prepared to rearrange their schedules so they can fit in a widowers' support group at a local hospital. Some people really love the support they receive by going to a cancer support group such as Gilda's Club. Or perhaps the comfort you're looking for may be found with a fitness group training together every few days to do a breast cancer walk for charity.

Other people can play such an important role in healing both your physical and emotional self. I have seen again and again how powerful a little "reaching out" has been for me. And I have felt privileged to offer help to others who may find what they're looking for in me.

Can you renew someone else's hope or light a little fire of encouragement inside another person on the journey from illness to health? I believe with all my heart that you can—and I hope with all my heart that you will.

> *I am a little pencil in the hand of a writing God who is sending a love letter to the world.*
> —Mother Teresa

Heavenly Lemon Cream

What better way to say thank you to a friend or family member who pitches in without being asked than to offer a dish of this truly luscious dessert? Such support deserves a reward!

❄ Serves 4

    1 (4-serving) package JELL-O sugar-free instant vanilla pudding mix
    1 (4-serving) package JELL-O sugar-free lemon gelatin
    ⅔ cup Carnation Nonfat Dry Milk Powder
    1 cup Diet Mountain Dew
    ½ cup Land O Lakes no-fat sour cream
    ½ cup Cool Whip Free

In a large bowl, combine dry pudding mix, dry gelatin, dry milk powder, and Diet Mountain Dew. Mix well using a wire whisk. Blend in sour cream and Cool Whip Free. Evenly spoon mixture into 4 dessert dishes. Refrigerate for at least 15 minutes.

Each serving equals:

HE: ½ Fat-Free Milk • 1 Slider • 5 Optional Calories

104　Calories • 0 gm　Fat • 6 gm　Protein • 20 gm　Carbohydrate • 282 mg Sodium • 170 mg Calcium • 0 gm Fiber

DIABETIC EXCHANGES: 1 Starch/Carbohydrate • ½ Fat-Free Milk

(from: *The Open Road Cookbook*)

Recipes for Comfort

Sad soul, take comfort, nor forget
That sunrise never failed us yet.
—Celia Thaxter

If I asked you to answer without thinking much about it, what would you say is your idea of comfort? You might blurt out, "A cup of cocoa on a cold night," or "Curled up in a favorite chair with a sleeping cat on my lap." Or you might say, "A hug that squeezes the stuffing out of me" or even "Knowing I have enough money in the bank to cover my bills this month."

Comfort means different things to each of us, and at no time in our lives are we hungrier or more full of longing for real, heartfelt comfort than when we're coping with a life-threatening illness or grieving after a personal tragedy.

Taking comfort, allowing ourselves to indulge in a kind of emotional or physical warmth without guilt, is a powerful tool for healing what ails us. But getting in touch with what really delivers the kind of comfort that soothes and relieves pain (the psychological and spiritual as well as the kind that stiffens our joints) takes practice—and a kind of awareness of what makes us feel truly good.

Here I have gathered together ingredients for comfort, the soul-deep kind that offer not only consolation but also a sense that, in the midst of difficult days, something will ease your sorrow or fear.

God knew we needed Duke before we did.

His warm brown eyes easily captured Cliff and me right from the beginning, and ever since my cancer diagnosis he's been a godsend to both of us. He's a perfect combination of golden and Labrador retriever, which to me says he gives more than he gets! When we're a little on the lonely side, he knows it—and he comes over and lets us just pet our worries away.

In the summer of 2001, before my symptoms started, we went to Ohio, where I was doing cooking demonstrations at a farm show. We put out enough food and water for our two cats, Jeff and Jason, and gave them the run of the house for the three days that we were going to be gone. I even said to Cliff as we got ready to leave, "It's a good thing we just have cats, isn't it? Because as much as we are gone, how could we ever take care of a dog?"

Well, while we were in Ohio, somebody dumped Duke off on our land. We figured they must have been leaving town, didn't want the dog anymore, and just drove out into the country and left him. When Duke showed up, Julia (my assistant Gina's daughter, who waters our plants while we're away) felt sorry for him and gave him something to drink and eat, so he just hung around. Maybe he was waiting for whoever dropped him off to come back and get him.

When we returned home, there he was waiting for *us*. At first, we thought, oh, no, we can't have a dog, but then he looked at us with those beautiful brown eyes, and we looked at each other and smiled.

It was Cliff who suggested calling him Duke. I said, "If I call him, and he comes, that will be it." So I called "Duke!" and he was right there, as if it had always been his name.

Well, we got him a dog bowl and bought him a doghouse and placed it under a shade tree. At first, he'd stay with us for a day or two and then be gone for a little bit. I think that he was still looking for the people who dropped him off.

I invited my grandkids over for the weekend and told them we had a new dog. But when they arrived, Duke wasn't here. Later that night, though, he came home, and they fell in love with him. But the next morning he was gone again.

That night, we took the boys to the drive-in theater up the road from us. We were sitting on lawn chairs in front of the car while the kids played nearby. The stars started to come out.

"Look Grandma," Zach said. "Let's make a wish."

I said, "All right. Let's say a prayer to God that if Duke is to be our dog, he'll be there when we get home." So the boys and I said a prayer and then watched the movie. And when we got home, there was Duke waiting for us.

As winter arrived in Iowa and the temperatures plummeted, Cliff thought it was too cold for Duke out in the doghouse. So we put him in the garage. But then it got so awfully cold in February that I wanted to bring him into the house.

Cliff kept saying no. But on one particularly bitter night, Cliff decided to put him in the laundry room when he went to bed.

That was just the beginning. Now he is 100 percent house dog, and he is the best-trained dog—ever. (Okay, maybe I'm prejudiced, but I know how good he is!) We didn't even have to train him—he just seemed to know what to do.

We can't even imagine what our lives would be like without him; he's that special. Now, if we have to go away somewhere for more than a day, we try to take our motor home so Duke can travel with us. And if we're going somewhere without the motor home, we always check to see if the place we're staying allows dogs.

Duke isn't just good company. He seems to know when I'm having a difficult time or a down day, and he doesn't want to let me out of his sight. He's amazingly sensitive to my moods, and he has a powerful healing effect on me. When he curls up next to me, I feel my heartbeat slowing down to a peaceful calm, and I know my blood pressure must be heading downward as well.

Dogs are not our whole life, but they make our lives whole.
—Roger Caras

Is there a Duke in your life, an animal that provides unconditional love and an endless source of comfort when nothing else seems to do the trick? I hope so! I never really understood just how important the affection and attention of a pet could be when you're so focused on staying well and remaining hopeful.

If I could spare him, Duke would make a fantastic therapy dog. I first heard about these "dogs with jobs" a few years ago. It seems that all over the country there are programs where dog owners volunteer their wonderful animals to provide what is called animal-assisted therapy (AAT), though I love some of the other names these programs have, including K-9 Candy Stripers and Prescription Pets!

They take dogs with really good temperaments and train them to be handled by patients in hospitals and nursing homes, people in schools for the mentally and physically disabled, and even correctional facilities. They bring such happiness and cheer to people who need something to hold and love; they often rekindle memories of pets they used to own; and they are remarkably successful in reaching adults and children who are socially withdrawn.

On the Therapy Dogs Inc. website (www.therapydogs. com), they tell it like it is: "Four-footed therapists give something medical science can't do, without the use of drugs. It has been clinically proven that through petting, touching, and talking with the animals, patients' blood pressure is lowered, stress is relieved, and depression is eased."

If you don't have a dog or cat, this could be a good time in your life to consider "taking the plunge." There are so many animals looking for good homes, and you might find yourself saving your own life by saving one of God's creatures as well! Sharing your life with a pet is good for the health and good for the heart—take it from me!

When I shared with a friend about how Duke is so good at knowing when I need him with me, she told me about a book called *Dogs That Know When Their Owners Are Coming Home* by biologist Rupert Sheldrake. After five years of research involving thousands of people who have pets and work with animals, Dr. Sheldrake proved what many pet owners already know: There is a strong connection between humans and animals that science can't explain or fully understand. It's the perfect book to put on your shelf next to another really good one called *Dogs Never Lie About Love* by Jeffrey Moussaieff Masson. It's full of stories that demonstrate what Cliff and I have learned in living with Duke: that dogs feel deep emotions, that they are honest, loving, sensitive, and intensely attached to their "people"!

I never tire of talking about Dukie—he's just the most perfect dog on the face of the earth. Dukie Lund. He knew his name from the first. He seemed to know us from the very beginning, and he quickly and completely became a loving, healing influence in my life. He gives us unconditional love and acceptance, and Cliff and I both love him with all our hearts.

And he returns that love. In fact, when we are both calling him, he doesn't know who to go to—so we go to him.

There are two ways to live your life. One is as though nothing is a miracle. The other is as though everything is a miracle.
—*Albert Einstein*

For me, there's almost no touch I love more than the brush of Duke's head against my leg, but I've also learned that this is a time for seeking out the human touch as a source of comfort and healing. I was so fortunate not to lose my hair while taking chemo, and I've found a more intense pleasure than in the past in having my hair cared for by a professional beautician.

It's a totally different experience to wash your own hair in the shower than it is to lie back and have strong, sure hands suds up your hair and massage your scalp with a fragrant shampoo, then gently dry it with a towel (that you don't have to wash!). I find getting my hair done so relaxing, even more so now that I've been undergoing treatment for my breast cancer.

If you're not a beauty parlor person, how about giving yourself the gift of a massage? Even if you've never had one, I hope you'll consider calling your local sports club or YMCA to treat yourself for a half hour or hour of rubbing, kneading, and manipulating your muscles. There are some massage therapists with experience working with patients undergoing cancer treatment, so if you'd rather work with one of them, ask the nurses where you're being treated for a recommendation. (If they don't know of someone, they can refer you to the hospital's physical therapy department.)

What feels good is good for you. Some breast cancer survivors I've spoken with are dedicated yoga enthusiasts. One told me, "It puts me back in touch with my body, after the mastectomy made me feel as if it wasn't quite me anymore."

And if none of these suggestions feels right for you, perhaps you'll want to make a commitment just to take better care of yourself. Treat yourself to a new body lotion that your post-treatment sense of smell finds appealing; maybe a foot rub (by your spouse or a friend) using cooling peppermint foot lotion will be just the thing to help you restore circulation in extremities that have grown a bit numb.

Only you can decide what kind of physical comfort will improve the quality of your life. I hope you'll choose to make the effort to find just what that might be for you!

※

Sometimes, comfort and inspiration are often no further away than your Sunday newspaper, and it was in there I discovered this beautiful essay by Alma Gaul, which ran in our local *Quad City Times*. It serves to remind us in just a few hundred words how precious life is—and how, when we pay attention to the smallest details of that life, we receive extraordinary consolation and solace.

REFLECTING ON THE WONDERS OF THE WORLD

As we race through summer with Bix [a Davenport, Iowa, jazz festival and road race in honor of Bix Beiderbecke] and trips and projects and practice, it's important to stop now and then and think about what we're doing and who we are.

Ideally, we would do this every day.

Ideally, we would set aside time in every day to be by ourselves, in quiet, to examine our lives to make sure they are being lived with purpose, with overarching goals, with gratitude for being.

Too often, this doesn't happen. We're too busy running from here to there, living from one list to the next, getting everything done.

And maybe all those things—running, lists, getting things done—really *do* add up to the kinds of lives we want to lead, even if we don't take time for examination.

Still, it never hurts to be a little more thoughtful, so that we are living with all the fullness and awareness we are capable of, that we are as joyous as possible, given the particular cards we've been dealt.

Where to start, though? Sometimes it helps to have a springboard—an idea to launch us into the pool of thought. Some time back I ran across an Internet communication that was a springboard for me. I don't know who wrote this, but they were smart:

"A group of students was asked to list what they thought were the present Seven Wonders of the World. Though there was some disagreement, the following got the most votes:

1. Egypt's Great Pyramids
2. Taj Mahal
3. Grand Canyon
4. Panama Canal

5. Empire State Building
6. St. Peter's Basilica
7. China's Great Wall

While gathering the votes, the teacher noted that one quiet student hadn't turned in her paper yet. So she asked the girl if she was having trouble with her list.

The girl replied, "Yes, a little. I couldn't quite make up my mind because there are so many."

The teacher said, "Well, tell us what you have and maybe we can help."

The girl hesitated, then read, "I think the Seven Wonders of the World are:

1. "To touch
2. To taste
3. To see
4. To hear."

She hesitated a little, then added,

5. "To feel
6. To laugh
7. And to love."

The room was full of silence.

Those things we overlook as simple and "ordinary" are truly wondrous. A gentle reminder that the most precious things in life cannot be bought . . .

Something to contemplate in our quest for full and joyous lives.

Alma's column reminded me that life is full of these everyday miracles, a million and one opportunities to experience God's blessings. Like many people, I've often spent most of my waking hours engaged in activity instead of contemplation, though my habit of getting up before dawn has helped me carve out a little time every day to commune with the Lord and to reflect on His many gifts.

Yet I was inspired by this chance encounter with Alma's newspaper piece to focus my heart and mind on each of that young girl's "wonders" and to experience for myself how truly extraordinary they can be.

To Touch

Are we in such a hurry as we move through our lives that we've let ourselves lose contact with the marvelous world around us? Each day, we experience so many sensations through our fingers and hands, through every inch of our skin, but do we stop to notice each individual feeling?

- Each hot, sharp prickle as the spray of the shower prods my flesh into wakefulness in the early morning hours . . .

- The smooth, cool, hard shape of a piece of antique carnival glass in my hand as I pick it up to dust it . . .

- The delicate, soft, sensual touch of a flower petal warmed by the sun so it almost feels like a loved one's cheek . . .

- The silky feel of a sweet little baby's bottom, which is absolutely irresistible to a grandmother's hand . . .

- The wonderful variety of textures I can experience simply by picking up different pieces of fruit—the bumpy skin of a fresh orange, the ready-to-burst feel of a ripe plum, the dry-smooth touch of a perfectly red apple . . .

Today I promise myself to pay attention to everything and anything that touches me. I will notice it all, from the firm but springy ground under my feet to the tender touch of gently falling rain. I will be touched by the world and touch it back!

To Taste

I saw a headline on the web that said that schoolchildren were given less than thirty minutes to eat their lunch, and that some days it was more like fifteen or less. How sad that already they're learning what too many adults know—to eat without tasting, to consume without using their senses to truly enjoy the food that nourishes them. Will we lose the ability—and the joy—of tasting?

- The succulent sensation of the very first bite of a juicy piece of chicken at a barbecue . . .

- The silken slide of a glass of cold milk poured down my throat on a hot summer's day . . .

- The wonderful rush of sweetness as I sink my teeth into a perfect peach picked right off my tree . . .

- The tickle of tiny bubbles on the tongue as I sip a chilled glass of my favorite Diet Dew after working in the garden . . .

- The rich blend of flavors and creamy smoothness in a piece of one of my healthy cheesecakes . . .

Today I will savor each mouthful that passes my lips and pause for a moment to marvel at the gift of taste. Even though my cancer treatment has occasionally altered this treasured sense, I can still enjoy sweet and sour, salty and tangy. I will taste all that the world has to offer and give thanks for being nourished by my food.

To See

We open our eyes as we awaken every morning, but so often we do not really look at the world around us, take it all in as if seeing it with new eyes. Yet each new day shows us something that we've never really seen before—if we will but only gaze at our environment and let it touch us. Did a marvel pass you by today without you giving it a second glance?

- The astonishing hues in just one fragile flower, from the palest ivory to the deepest, darkest purple of the heart of a petunia . . .

- The unexpected beauty of a young child's innocent pleasure in a game of hopscotch or tag . . .

- The thrilling speed and grace of a red-tailed hawk as it swoops and dives over a field of corn . . .

- The surprise of admiring a reflection in the darkened window of a store and wondering who that attractive person may be . . .

- Discovering something new about yourself in the mirror that pleases and intrigues you . . .

Today I will use my eyes to bring the outside into me. I will not only look but also see, and not only see, but also seek to understand what I view. I will stop to see what's beautiful and good instead of only noticing what's standing in my way or slowing me down.

To Hear

Have you shut your ears to some of life's sweetest sounds because the world has become too noisy, too much of a distraction? Have you stopped listening to the hum and hubbub all around you because you are caught up in the echoes in your own head? Perhaps it is time to open what's been closed and start to hear what the universe is telling you.

- The whirring, rhythmic hum of a cloud of bees, feeding on the nectar in your garden . . .

- The high, sharp whistle of a train fading into the distance as its *chug-chugging* engine moves along the railroad track . . .

- The yearning song of an unseen bird who awakens you at 3 A.M. with a plaintive cry for its mate . . .

- The sweet, loud giggles of a trio of schoolgirls sharing the secrets of their first crushes on boys . . .

- An unexpected burst of country music coming from a trucker's radio as his big rig rumbles by . . .

Today I will listen to the melody of the world around me, hearing its themes and moving to its beat. I recall the line from the musical *Oklahoma!* that "all the sounds of the earth are like music," and I will make a point of singing along!

To Feel

Some emotions are uncomfortable, and so many people rush along without reflecting on or reacting to the people and events in their lives. But when we turn off the switch of feelings, we limit ourselves to a much narrower world of experience. It may seem safer to hurry past the situations that make us feel sad or lonely or disappointed, but are we missing out on feeling the highs in our lives?

- Watching what my mother used to call a "seven-handkerchief-picture" and having a good cry over the problems of the people on the screen . . .

- Having a lemonade at the coffee shop when all the high school kids pile in, and feeling a momentary twinge at how young they are—and you aren't anymore . . .

- Feeling grateful for the wisdom that comes with experience and a little relief that you'll never have to repeat the struggles the young are just starting to experience . . .

- Walking through your house at dawn and enjoying a quiet sense of pride about how you've made it yours . . .

- Sitting alone on a park bench after a solitary walk because you couldn't get anyone else to come with you—and discovering that when God is present, you are never alone . . .

Today I will let myself feel all of the emotions, from sorrow to joy and everything in between. The more deeply I experience my life, the richer my memories and my relationships will be. Whether my heart beats fast with excitement or gently in moments of calm and relaxation, I will pay attention to all that my senses bring to me and revel in the miracle that is my life.

To Laugh

As you grow older and face the challenges of aging or illness, it can become a little harder to grin at a joke or shake with the giggles over a comedian's pratfall on television. But we cannot allow ourselves to surrender to a world that is humorless and dry—it's bad for your health, as Norman Cousins and others have written. Laughter heals, and it also lightens our burdens, so we've really got to "find the funny" in our lives.

- Paging through old photo albums and shuddering a little at some of the styles we wore "back then" . . .

- Cleaning out the refrigerator and discovering a sealed container of "who knows what?" in the very back . . .

- Repeating "Who's there?" a hundred times when your grandson keeps saying, "Knock, knock!"

- Pulling a baking pan out of the oven and shaking your head at the weird color or shape of the dish being tested . . .

- Catching a glimpse of yourself in the mirror after a couple of hours of gardening and discovering that you're caked with dirt from head to toe . . .

Today I will smile instead of frown when something ridiculous occurs. (Remember, it takes fewer muscles to smile!) I will see the humor in domestic disasters, I will laugh at myself at least once, and if I can't find something to grin about, I'll put a silly movie on the DVD and howl at the funny parts!

To Love

Love is more than the seventh wonder of the world. It's the greatest gift we have, and the one we probably take most for granted on any given day. But paying attention to what love is and can be enriches our lives beyond measure.

- The briefest caress—a pat on the back, a touch on the arm—sends a silent message that love is all around . . .

- A few words of affection, or an unexpected phone call to say you're thinking of someone, gives love a voice . . .

- Letting a loved one know what you're feeling, even if you're scared or sad, is a gift of loving trust . . .

- Choose to act in love, by making his favorite lunch or fixing the old jeans you'd rather he threw out . . .

- Meditate on the power of love by closing your eyes and filling your heart with memories . . .

Today I will tell the people I love just how much and in what ways I love them. I will love what's good about them and I will love what I may want to change about them. Love is a paintbrush that brings color and light to our lives. If you feel there isn't enough love in your life, begin by loving yourself and sharing yourself with others. Love has an amazing way of coming back to you when you do.

Each day we are blessed with the ability to touch, to taste, to see, to hear, to feel, to laugh, and to love, and those blessings are a precious gift, a comfort in tough times. I no longer take for granted the moist kisses my grandchildren plant on my face. I no longer consider ordinary the beautiful sunrise and sunset that begins and ends the days of my life. And I wouldn't think of turning down a pleasant ride in the country with Cliff by my side. Each and every day that I am blessed with these "ordinary things," these true wonders, I offer a prayer of thankfulness to God!

God gave you a gift of 86,400 seconds today. Have you used one to say "thank you"?

—William A. Ward

Double Layer Lemon Dessert

Some people say that nearly all of my recipes are their idea of "comfort food," but this one truly is! It's smooth, creamy, and oh-so-soothing after a rough day.

❊ Serves 8

12 (2½-inch) graham cracker squares

2 (4-serving) packages JELL-O sugar-free lemon gelatin

1 (4-serving) package JELL-O sugar-free vanilla cook-and-serve pudding mix

2½ cups water

1 (4-serving) package JELL-O sugar-free instant vanilla pudding mix

⅔ cup Carnation Nonfat Dry Milk Powder

¾ cup Cool Whip Free

1 teaspoon coconut extract

2 tablespoons flaked coconut

Evenly arrange 10 graham cracker squares in an 11-by-7-inch biscuit pan. In a medium saucepan, combine 1 package dry gelatin, dry cook-and-serve pudding mix, and 1½ cups water. Cook over medium heat until mixture thickens and starts to boil, stirring often. Remove from heat and allow to cool 2 to 3 minutes. Pour pudding mixture evenly over graham crackers. Refrigerate for at least 30 minutes. In a medium bowl, combine remaining 1 package dry gelatin, dry instant pudding mix, dry milk powder, and remaining 1 cup water. Mix well using a wire whisk. Blend in Cool Whip Free and coconut extract. Spread mixture evenly over set lemon layer. Finely crush remaining 2 graham crackers. In a small bowl, combine cracker crumbs and coconut. Evenly sprinkle mixture over top. Refrigerate for at least 15 minutes. Cut into 8 servings.

Each serving equals:

HE: ½ Bread • ¼ Fat-Free Milk • ½ Slider • 7 Optional Calories

89 Calories • 1 gm Fat • 4 gm Protein • 16 gm Carbohydrate • 348 mg Sodium • 69 mg Calcium • 0 gm Fiber

DIABETIC EXCHANGES: 1 Starch/Carbohydrate

(from: *Diabetic Desserts Cookbook*)

Recipes for Faith

Faith is putting all your eggs in God's basket, then counting your blessings before they hatch.
                    —Ramona C. Carroll

If there is ever a time to lose your faith or feel it become terribly fragile and vulnerable, it's when you first hear terrible news or a frightening prognosis.

At first, you can't believe that something terrible could happen to someone who has done her best, helped others, worshipped regularly, and tried to live a life that was pleasing to the Lord.

And yet it does happen, just as so many before you have had their faith tested by painful events. The Bible is filled with stories of people who were asked to suffer, and so many of the lessons we draw from it remind us that faith means believing in what we cannot see. Sustaining that belief in the moments when we fear God has abandoned us is the true test of our love.

We take so much in our lives on faith.

A baker puts a loaf of dough into the oven with a firm belief that heat and yeast and moisture will somehow come together and make bread.

A man and a woman express their love, and nine months later, in a mystery and miracle that is at least one part faith, a child is born of that love.

The seasons change, the sun comes up, and life goes on—all of these taken on faith. Oh, of course we know that science plays a major role in all of this, but there's always just a little bit of the unknown that is eternal, divine, beyond our complete control.

I discovered in these past few years that you need an extra added serving of faith when dealing with a diagnosis of cancer. Or how would we ever make our peace with the knowledge that treating the disease requires walking a very fine line between life and death?

Chemotherapy, after all, is the deliberate introduction of a poisonous substance into our bodies, delivered in carefully measured doses designed to kill the cancer cells without also hurting the normal ones. How do we dare do this?

We have to have faith.

Faith in our doctors, whose advice we depend on for our return to good health.

Faith in the research of unknown scientists, whose endless hours of work so often ends in frustration and failure.

Faith in our friends and families, who support us through sickness and despair, through a thousand little struggles to find the "new normal."

Faith in ourselves, that we will find the courage and endurance it takes to survive an illness with a terrifying prognosis.

And of course faith in the Lord, into whose hands we give our lives and hope that He will grant us all the tomorrows we want to see.

Now faith is being sure of what we hope for and certain of what we do not see.

—Hebrews 11:1

We fix our eyes not on what is seen but on what is unseen. For what is seen is temporary but what is unseen is eternal.

—2 Corinthians 4:18

The Bible is filled with reminders of what faith is and is not. But in times of crises it may be hard to have faith in God's plan. It is only natural to ask, "God, why me?" Of course, I can understand how many people might cry out, "Lord, I've tried to live my life in a righteous way, so why have you forsaken me?"

When I first heard the words "*You have cancer,*" I felt my body freeze in a kind of shock, but I also felt myself move a tiny step closer to the Lord. Cancer didn't make me doubt my faith in God; instead, it gave me a better reason to run to His arms.

Over time, I've come to look at getting cancer as a sort of

blessing, as part of my "assignment" here on this earth. Maybe I'm supposed to use what I learn to inform other people about this rare form of cancer, or maybe God wanted me to have a wake-up call—to make some life changes that are good for me and my family at this time in our lives.

The truth, of course, is that I don't know.

None of us do.

But if we can have faith that what happens to us may have a purpose, we are just better equipped to face it and come through.

❖

To be a gardener, as I have been all my life, you have to begin with faith, because so much of what happens there is unseen—at least for a while. You need to have a vision of what you hope to see, and then you begin working toward making that vision a reality. But unlike many occupations, such as writing a book or building a house, you don't have hands-on control over everything that develops.

Your faith that the seeds you plant will germinate is not unlike the faith a cook must have when placing her cake pan into the oven: you've provided the ingredients, you've got a source of heat—but what actually happens is not in your hands, but in God's. (Of course, there is kitchen chemistry involved, too!)

The same is true when you are coping with a medical crisis. If you don't have faith in the treatment you're given, if you don't envision the good health you hope to see, it's less likely that your body will respond as well as you hope. Researchers have observed that patients who believe in the potential of their medicines generally do better than those who are suffused with doubt and despair. In some studies, patients who were given a placebo—a pill that did not contain the actual healing ingredients—reacted as if they had received the real thing. The power of their faith made it possible for them to improve medically even without taking the drug being studied.

❋

A friend wrote to me, some months before my diagnosis, and shared a homily she'd heard given in an Episcopal church in the South Bronx, a very impoverished area of New York City. The priest was a woman who'd worked as a lawyer much of her life, someone who'd found a calling to the church after doing volunteer work for a local tenants' organization. "God plans ahead," the priest said. "Everything you've done up to this moment has prepared you for what lies ahead."

Can you take that statement on faith?

Can you accept it when you've been asked to bear a cross of some kind and believe that your suffering has value?

Are you willing to trust in God and follow a new path that veers from the one you've been taking for so long?

All good questions, and not easily answered.

Not every crisis is about life and death, but so many times in our lives, we're faced with uncomfortable changes and shattered dreams of one kind or another. How we meet our destiny can be a gift to God, but first we have to see clearly what is being asked of us.

I like to say that "Flowers can't grow in the dark, they need the sunshine." It's the same with how we live our lives. If we're cursing our fate and blaming God, we can't concentrate on growing in the sunshine. It's as if we're keeping the clouds overhead by being unable to have faith in what God has planned for us.

We always have the choice of how to react to unexpected trouble, to crises that force us to stop and regroup.

In 2002, my son Tom experienced a serious crisis at his job. Without notice, Tom and a thousand other employees at his company received calls telling them not to report to work the next morning. In the aftermath of this shocking news, Tom wrote to one of his former colleagues in an attempt to understand the seeming randomness of this situation, which had such an enormous impact on so many lives. I asked him to share his letter with us here.

TURNING ON FLASHLIGHTS

Just because we can only see and experience events with our limited senses doesn't mean there's no order. My favorite analogy for explaining this is to imagine that you find yourself in a pitch-dark room with only a small flashlight.

When you turn on the flashlight, you can only "see" a very limited area of the floor at any one time—call it "the present." As you move around the room—as you experience more places—you may remember the spots where you were—the past—even though you can no longer see them.

And wherever you decide to focus your light next is the future. You can't see that place yet, but it's there waiting for you. No matter what direction it "feels" like you're wandering in, you still end up in the same room that you were "put" in, and that you're supposed to be in.

Just like in life, you are not alone in the dark room. There are others wandering about with their own flashlights. From time to time, your lighted areas connect. You're both at the same place and time in your lives.

The more people there are in the room shining their lights, the more we are collectively gaining "knowledge" about this mysterious room. People explore in different parts of this universe and then come back periodically to share the experiences of their discoveries.

Meanwhile, the master architect of this magnificent place sits perched up in the balcony overlooking the action. Like a proud parent watching his children from a distance as the child discovers the wonders of the universe, He enthusiastically and lovingly observes us down here exploring.

While none of us can see Him directly, we catch glimpses and clues in what we find here that there is a guiding hand, and that we didn't get there by chance. The people hear "silent whispers of gentle persuasion" to go this way or that way. Some they act upon. Other times, they don't. These whispers are not voices we hear with our ears, but they're there nonetheless.

Usually the evidence for order in this seeming chaos comes

and goes so rapidly and so frequently that we dismiss it as happenstance or coincidence. It doesn't follow us as we move to a different spot, yet for a short time afterward we remember it. Then it fades.

Some other evidence comes into our view, and then it passes. And so it goes until at some point we find ourselves at the bottom of the stairs to the balcony. It's the end of the wandering. We go upstairs, where the true beauty of the entire view is revealed before our eyes. It still remains beyond our understanding at that point—how it all works—as we stare in awe, but we can finally see and understand the effects of all of the steps we took as we wandered about—and how they had an impact on others.

When I take the time to stop pushing "forward," this is what I imagine. I do not believe in luck or chance. As a person with an education in statistics, you would think that I do. But, actually, random variability, or noise, is just something we humans attach to unforeseen variables—when our "flashlights" aren't big enough to see the whole picture, if we're looking in the wrong direction, or when the object spreads out too far.

OK, I'll stop now. Back to the world we can observe . . .

> *A little faith will bring your soul to heaven,*
> *but a lot of faith will bring heaven to your soul.*
> —*Author Unknown*

Faith gets tested.

I've learned this firsthand during my journey in search of health and on the road to remission.

In the summer of 2003, I was sailing along so well. Every time I'd go in for my regular appointment, my doctor would just be amazed at how well I was doing. It was wonderful.

Soon, it was time to go off one chemo protocol and start another one. About six weeks into the new chemo, I felt a lump under my arm again, and everything came to a screeching halt.

For almost a year and a half, it had been such smooth sailing, beyond what anyone in the medical profession could have predicted for me. I was still doing everything the same—following my doctors' instructions, thinking positively, turning it over to God—and yet here the cancer had started in again with a vengeance.

I could have let it send me into despair, thinking it was the beginning of the end. But I didn't want to go there. I didn't want to shake my fist at heaven and yell, *I'm doing my part, how come You're not doing Yours?*

Instead, I just turned my crisis over to God and kept going. It was the right decision for me. With a new protocol and God's blessing, we again got the cancer under control!

I think these bumps in the road are there to teach us something. What did I learn this time around? When we combine the best medical advancements available to us with prayer, we're doing all we can. Prayer alone probably isn't going to heal us, and medicine alone may or may not do enough, but when we combine them and put ourselves in God's hands, I believe we'll be healed one way or another. The physical ailment may subside, but if we don't overcome it, we'll be rejoicing in heaven where there will be no pain.

I feel that I've been so lucky on this journey. Everyone I've met has just been wonderful. I haven't encountered any medical people who didn't reach out and do anything and everything they could to make things easier for me. I like to say, When we look for the good in people, we find it.

Some of them don't know they're reaching out that little extra but they are. Their generosity and willingness to support me every step of the way has certainly reinforced my faith that people are, by nature, good. Almost everyone in times of need is going to reach out and help and not expect something back. When people know a fellow human being needs help, they really respond.

Faith is taking the first step even when you don't see the whole staircase.

—*Dr. Martin Luther King, Jr.*

Around the time of my fifty-eighth birthday, when I was focusing on celebrating life and sustaining my faith, I received this beautiful cyberessay, which echoed exactly what I was feeling.

THE YELLOW ROSES

I walked into the grocery store not particularly interested in buying groceries. I wasn't hungry. The pain of losing my husband of seven years was still too raw. And this grocery store held so many sweet memories. He often came with me and almost every time he'd pretend to go off and look for something special. I knew what he was up to. I'd always spot him walking down the aisle with three yellow roses in his hands. He knew I loved yellow roses.

With a heart filled with grief, I only wanted to buy my few items and leave, but even grocery shopping was different since he had passed on. Shopping for one took time, a little more thought than it had for two. Standing by the meat, I searched for the perfect small steak and remembered how he loved his steak. Suddenly a woman came beside me. She was blonde, slim, and lovely in a soft green pantsuit. I watched as she picked up a large pack of T-bones, dropped them into her basket, hesitated, and then put them back in the display. She turned to go and once again reached for the pack of steaks. She saw me watching her and she smiled. "My husband loves T-bones, but honestly, at these prices, I don't know."

I swallowed the emotion down my throat and met her pale blue eyes. "My husband passed away eight days ago," I told her. Glancing at the package in her hands, I fought to control the tremble in my voice. "Buy him the steaks. And cherish every moment you have together." She shook her head and I saw the emotion in her eyes as she placed the package in her basket and wheeled away.

I turned and pushed my cart across the length of the store to the dairy products. There I stood, trying to decide which size milk I should buy. Quart, I finally decided and moved on to the ice cream. If nothing else, I could always fix myself an ice cream cone. I placed the ice cream in my cart and looked down the aisle toward the front. I saw first the green pantsuit, then recognized the pretty lady coming toward me. In her arms she carried a package. On her face was the brightest smile I had ever seen. I would swear a soft halo encircled her blonde hair as she kept walking toward me, her eyes holding mine.

As she came closer, I knew what she held and tears began misting in my eyes. "These are for you," she said as she placed three beautiful long-stemmed yellow roses in my arms. "When you go through the line, they know these are already paid for," she said. Then, she leaned over and placed a gentle kiss on my cheek, then smiled again. I wanted to tell her what she'd done, what the roses meant to me, but I was still unable to speak, I watched as she walked away as tears clouded my vision. I looked down at the beautiful roses nestled in the green tissue wrapping and found it almost unreal. How did she know? Suddenly the answer seemed clear. I wasn't alone. "Oh, you haven't forgotten me have you?" I whispered with tears in my eyes. He was still with me and she was his angel. Every day be thankful for what you have and who you are.

—Anonymous

Some of you will read this and might think it's about death, while others will understand that with God's help we can get on in life no matter what's thrown our way. Maybe you never dreamed that you'd be battling cancer or coping with a potentially fatal disease.

I never did. But I am, and I'll continue to fight it with all my might for as long as I can. For that very reason, each and every birthday that I celebrate will be one more reason to rejoice!

Prayer is the key to heaven, but faith unlocks the door.
—Samuel T. Scott

Scrumptious Surprise Lemon Pie

When I first started working my "Healthy Exchanges" magic on rich desserts, I needed to believe that such healthy transformations were not only possible but surprisingly easy to perform. I had faith then that I could do it, and all these years later, I renew my faith each and every day.

❄ Serves 8

1 (8-ounce) package Philadelphia fat-free cream cheese

2 tablespoons Splenda Granular

1 teaspoon vanilla extract

1 cup Cool Whip Lite

1 (6-ounce) Keebler shortbread pie-crust

¼ cup chopped pecans

1 (4-serving) package JELL-O sugar-free instant vanilla pudding mix

1 (4-serving) package JELL-O sugar-free lemon gelatin

⅔ cup Carnation Nonfat Dry Milk Powder

1⅓ cups water

In a large bowl, stir cream cheese with a sturdy spoon until soft. Add Splenda, vanilla extract, and ¼ cup Cool Whip Lite. Mix well to combine. Spread mixture evenly into piecrust. Sprinkle pecans evenly over cream cheese mixture. In a medium bowl, combine dry pudding mix, dry gelatin, dry milk powder, and water. Mix well using a wire whisk. Spread pudding mixture evenly over pecans. Spread remaining ¾ cup Cool Whip Lite evenly over top. Refrigerate for at least 2 hours. Cut into 8 servings.

Each serving equals:

HE: ½ Bread • ½ Fat • ½ Protein • ¼ Fat-Free Milk • 1 Slider • 9 Optional Calories

208 Calories • 8 gm Fat • 8 gm Protein • 26 gm Carbohydrate • 424 mg Sodium • 1 gm Fiber

DIABETIC EXCHANGES: 1½ Starch • 1 Fat. ½ Meat

(from: *The Diabetic's Healthy Exchanges Cookbook*)

Recipes for Joy

The kiss of the sun for pardon,
The song of the birds for mirth,
One is nearer God's heart in a garden
Than anywhere else on earth.
—Dorothy Frances Gurney, "Garden Thoughts"

What is joy? Can you describe the feeling—and can you remember the times of your life when your entire being was filled with that beautiful, intense happiness?

Without the capacity to experience joy, we move through our lives like sturdy robots, going through the motions but never recognizing those miraculous, precious moments when we know why we're on this earth. For many of us, joy comes in those sweet seconds when we feel God's love, or when we sense what His purpose is for us. But there are other joyful times—some we recognize because we expect them to occur, such as when a baby first smiles or a daughter says "I do";

others are easy to miss but rare and wonderful all the same—the rush of pleasure after playing a song on the piano as well as you ever could, the feeling of accomplishment when a child you're tutoring reads a page without stopping and grins at the end.

The first and most important ingredient in any "recipe" for joy is being alive in every moment, so that not a single joyous blink-of-an-eye is missed!

For me, joy begins in the garden—and always has. All my life, I have planted gardens and spent my happiest hours working in them, communing with the Lord and with His magnificent creations in nature. In these past couple of years, the time I've spent in my gardens has been a powerful part of my healing journey. The physical labor has been my best exercise, besides walking. The sensual pleasure of digging in the black dirt and inhaling the scents of my flowers has helped me remain positive through very difficult times. And the constant small joys produced by each and every growing thing continues to keep my spirits high in the face of serious illness.

I also grow my own herbs—what a blessing for any cook, to know she will always be able to prepare meals using her own harvest. My chives come up every year like clockwork, and my oregano never fails, nor does my thyme. There's parsley, rosemary, and lots of dill. Even if you don't have a little (or large) plot of land to plant, you can still grow delicious herbs in a window box or on your kitchen windowsill.

We also have a beautiful orchard, with dwarf fruit trees that give us the Lord's bounty in luscious abundance. Fruit trees reward the gardener twice—first, with a profusion of aromatic blossoms and then with those precious ripening fruits.

Most days, I have the energy to walk through my gardens and inhale the sweet scents of earth and grass, but even on days when my strength is low, I manage to enjoy the lovely fruits of our labor.

More than two dozen benches are set amidst the gardens all over our property. Whenever my son Tommy comes to visit, he looks around for any new garden "room" I've made since his last visit, and asks if I think I have enough places for people to sit yet.

I always say, "No, I don't, Tom, but I'm working on it." I need them all because I have a big family, lots of friends, and from time to time, invite groups to tour my gardens. But the best reason for this "extravagance" is that it gives me joy!

> *To cultivate a garden is to walk with God.*
> —Christian Nestell Bovee

Part of the joy I get from my gardens is the knowledge that they will live and flourish after I'm gone. But it's not only my legacy that will endure. Beside our backyard porch, I've planted my Heritage Park. Everything that's growing there is linked with love to our families and the past. Heritage Park is filled with all the types of flowers and shrubs that my mother or Cliff's mother grew in their gardens years ago. My children and grandchildren know the stories of how their ancestors grew these plants, and they'll be able to share those stories with their own children someday.

※

I love the look of more formal gardens, but I also revel in the unplanned variety of my Hillside Garden. It's filled with perennials, and it looks like a wildly colorful patchwork quilt. Whatever I had in my hand when I was digging a hole, that's what went in there.

I just started planting at one end, and then went over to the other end, working my way toward the center. When I finally "met in the middle," I told Cliff I knew exactly how those railroad workers felt when they finished building the Transcontinental Railroad.

To me, this garden is a perfect illustration of serendipity, which is defined as a stroke of luck, a way of making unexpected and fortunate discoveries. So much that happens in our lives is unpredictable but delightful—a recipe that I thought would look and taste in one particular way turns out to be something very different, or a newsletter column I started to write that I thought would be about one thing and evolved into something I hadn't known at first I wanted to say. As the writer Tom Robbins once wrote, "Expect nothing. Be prepared for joy."

So much of science depends on this kind of serendipity, too. Some of the most important medical discoveries have occurred when the researchers were working on one thing that led to something entirely different but thrillingly lifesaving! Think of Sir Alexander Fleming, the British scientist who is credited with the discovery of penicillin, which has saved so many lives over the years. He was researching something else when by chance he noticed some mold that had developed on a plate containing bacteria. That mold was a crude form of what became known as penicillin!

As a cancer survivor who owes my continued survival to more than a few brilliant cancer researchers, I've seen that even scientists operate in just that way in the laboratory. Without specific expectations, they work with microbes invisible to the naked eye, but if and when they discover that these living things have powers they can learn to harness, the satisfaction is profound.

I may never "harness" the wild profusion of color and scent that covers my hillside, but I celebrate the glorious "accidents" and good fortune that provides me with such splendor!

※

Down by our walkout basement patio, off the lower level of our house, I've built my Garden of Hope and Healing. This garden is filled with perennials, shrubs, and plants that people gave me when I was first diagnosed with breast cancer. It's just turning into something very beautiful, and is a constant reminder that I'm not alone in my fight to survive this disease.

My gardens are not only for my enjoyment, of course—they're also places for my family to find peace and pleasure. Sharing their joy deepens my own, especially when my grandchildren pitch in. I was raised to believe that we are stewards of the land around us, that it is our duty and our delight to care for it during our lifetimes—and then to pass it on. My grandkids all understand my loving commitment to my gardens, and I firmly believe they will continue to sustain it all their lives.

※

Joy is personal, of course, and what delights me may fill you with dread or boredom. Take weeding, for example. Most people view it as a painful chore, something you do because you have to but certainly not a source of delight.

I may be one of the few people on earth who really does enjoy pulling weeds. There's a sense of satisfaction in it that I just can't quite describe. And because I don't use any pesticides, I need to make a real effort to keep the weeds from overrunning the place!

Sure, occasionally the weeds may get ahead of me, but I'm not going to get upset about it. Remember, I garden for the pleasure, not for the perfection.

※

For as long as I can remember, walking and riding my bike have energized and delighted me. Even on my busiest days, I've made time for some moderate exercise—and I didn't want a diagnosis of cancer to turn me into an invalid. I felt I needed my strength to keep up the fight.

But you don't always get what you want—at least, you may not get it the way you envision it. Oh, I still get out and do some walking every day, but not as far or as fast as I used to.

When Cliff is home from the road, he walks with me. But these days, gardening has become my exercise of choice.

That's something else I've had to accept, something that most people with cancer face. I've had to make peace with the fact that though I could once walk three or four miles without thinking about it, those days are over.

I am happy with one or two miles, because my energy isn't what it once was. I have to know my limitations—part of my "new normal"—and remember to rest when I need it. It's important to keep doing what you love, but just as I had to learn how to conserve my energy for what I wanted to do, you will discover how much physical activity is right for you. You don't want to overdo it, but you also don't want to baby yourself; you have to find the balance between what you *want* to do and what you *can* do now.

My gardens are my great joy, and they are also an expression of my deepest faith in God and the future. The seeds I plant grow unseen at first, just as faith does, but with time and prayer and His love, my garden grows into all it can be—and so do I.

I tell my family, The day I stop planning and planting is the day that they'd better start worrying about me. Until then, I express my joy and faith daily—and keep digging in the dirt!

The optimist sees the doughnut; the pessimist sees the hole.
—Author Unknown

Did I make you laugh, or at least smile, with my little doughnut joke? Good. Because the joy that comes from laughter is good for you! As every issue of *Reader's Digest* reminds us, "Laughter Is the Best Medicine."

Finding the "funny" in daily life is part of what gets us through the difficult and depressing realities that are a part of coping with cancer and other serious health challenges. You may surprise or even shock the people around you when you burst into giggles after knocking over a display of oranges in the supermarket or sliding off the sofa when you're taking an afternoon nap.

But that's just it—life is often silly or ridiculous, and instead of expressing annoyance at these little mix-ups or disasters, it's better to laugh.

And it's better to, as the song goes, "Ac-cent-uate the positive!"

A long time ago, I made the choice to try and live my life with a positive outlook, even when there are times when there isn't much to be positive about! Positive attitude may or may not add to the months or years of my life. But one thing I know for sure—it will definitely make whatever time I have left not only more enjoyable for me, but for those around me as well.

Yesterday's mail brought a note from a friend who quoted Helen Keller, a woman who managed to be positive enough to rise above the incredible challenges and disability of both blindness and deafness. "Character cannot be developed in ease and quiet," Keller wrote. "Only through experience of trial and suffering can the soul be strengthened, vision cleared, ambition inspired, and success achieved."

Alongside that thought-provoking quote was a reminder that

something positive often comes from struggling with a difficult situation, that only in the struggle to break free of the cocoon does a butterfly gain the strength to fly.

I never knew that.

But what a powerful argument for doing your best to prevail against difficult odds! You're building character, you're strengthening your soul—and you're learning how to fly.

※

Remaining positive when you're being treated for cancer isn't easy—but it makes a real difference, especially with all the ups and downs as your body reacts and responds to chemo and other treatments. I remember the day my oncologist said he was amazed at how well I was responding to my chemo protocol. Then he added that, even though I'd likely be on some form of chemo for the rest of my life, I could now consider my condition "chronic!"

What I also heard was what he *didn't* say: that I again have the strong possibility of a normal life span to look forward to! I couldn't wait to "share the joy" with the members of my inflammatory breast cancer website. Joy is increased when you share it with others—or at least it feels that way!

I remember when a new member of our "club" posted a message last year around Christmastime. This young mother of three children had just learned that she had IBC. She was hoping for any words of encouragement from someone else dealing with the disease. Was there any possibility that she might live to see her children grow into young adults? she asked.

I wrote back as soon as I could, hoping that my words might be just what she needed and wanted to hear:

"Dear ———: I was diagnosed with IBC in my left breast. By the time I knew what it was, it had already spread to my entire chest wall, to the outside breast skin, to every lymph node in my left armpit, and to several places in my bones. Today, I'm doing quite well and, in fact in my sixties, can hopefully look forward to seeing my eight grandchildren graduate from college.

"Right now, you are scared and you have every right to be. But if you find what works for you (not what works for the next person—but you!) you will find peace and acceptance, and along with that, you just might experience your own miracle, just as I am doing!"

She wrote back to say she felt encouraged by my story and by others shared on the website. Was it enough to help silence her fears and view her future more positively? Perhaps. As one of my own favorite inspirations comes from a book by A. L. Williams, *All You Can Do Is All You Can Do, But All You Can Do Is Enough!*

✻

I am reminded of the day I was getting my chemo treatment and noticed a man getting his at the same time. He was evidently on a brand-new protocol, which meant that the nurses had to double- and triple-check every step of the way. It was all going much more slowly than he would have liked.

He was getting upset with the nurse and complained aloud, "I should have been done two hours ago and here I am still in this chair." He was taking out all his frustration on the nurse, who I could see was almost in tears when she told him, "We'll get you out of here as soon as we can."

I promptly said to her, "You can take as long with me as you want. I don't care if I sit here all day long, because you're helping me keep on living so I can do the things I want to do. I don't begrudge you one minute of the time you have to take to check on me."

The man looked at me, somewhat sheepishly, and immediately stopped complaining. He went on with his chemo and I went on with mine. I don't always speak up like that, but his attitude got to me, and I just felt I had to say something.

It's true that I do look for the good in situations and people, and that I try to spot the silver linings in every cloud that blocks the sun. Living with cancer has made me zero in on what is precious; it's also shown me that it's hard to experience joy when you're shrouded in a cloud of negativity.

※

What else can you do to let joy in?

You can go back to the little pleasures that fell by the wayside in recent years, when life seemed too full for true leisure and work or family needs pushed your own needs to the back burner.

Do you ever take those little quizzes in women's magazines? When I'm in the beauty parlor waiting, I sometimes read through them, and one day this little quiz asked for a list of activities that were yours and yours alone. What did you love to do when it's just you for an hour or two?

After I made a mental list of mine, I was shocked to realize that I hadn't done any of the things on my list for way too long. I promised myself that that would change—and I started making time for what had always made me feel good.

Reading was first on my list, but for much of the last decade, I've been so busy working I almost gave up reading for pleasure. Now, I've been doing a lot more of it, just kicking back with a book and traveling to somewhere far, far away from here in both time and place.

So what if my floor needs dusting?

It can wait.

I'm going to read my book.

I cook for a living, but I also cook for pleasure. And, lucky for me, I have not become overly sensitive to cooking smells. Also, my taste for food hasn't been as affected as I feared it might be because of chemo, though sometimes I do get a metallic taste in my mouth.

So now I have an excellent excuse to invite lots of other opinions from my family and employees on the dishes I create. What was once almost solely about *my* taste buds has become a "family affair," a team operation in more ways than one. I try to give it a bit of a party atmosphere. Every day the ladies who work with me in our print shop come up to the house for lunch. Right alongside each dish there are sheets of paper for their comments about what they're eating. We talk, we laugh, they offer suggestions to make recipes tastier if needed, and I have grown to enjoy the give-and-take. Who knew?

※

Does all this talk about joy and positive attitude get you riled up? You're not alone. Recently, there was a discussion on my inflammatory breast cancer website about positive attitude. Someone had written to say, "Keep up your strength and your positive attitude," and one woman responded that she was getting a little tired of all this positive attitude stuff, saying that a positive attitude really doesn't save anyone's life. She added, "Think of all these good people who have died, and they had positive outlooks, and it didn't make a difference."

Well, I wrote back to her that I believe that for me it does. I've done my best to keep a positive attitude throughout my treatment and while it may not add measurable time to my life, I do feel it makes all the minutes of my life better for me and for all those around me.

Am I looking at this through rose-colored glasses? It might seem so, but this is just how I feel, even after I've been to the brink of death and back. I've had my cries, and I've had my ups and downs like everyone else, but I always try to look for something positive, and I almost always find it.

A lively discussion ensued on the website. Lots of people joined in, and most seconded what I had said. If a positive attitude was all it took, people wouldn't be dying right and left—

and they are. But a positive attitude does make the life we have, those precious weeks and months and years, more enjoyable.

Besides, there have been studies over the years that suggest that optimism, trying to make the best of every situation, actually can have a positive effect on your health. Who knows, maybe if I didn't have such a positive attitude *before* I was diagnosed with cancer, I wouldn't have made it through those scary first few months!

❖

You're going to have good days and bad ones. You're going to get your hopes up about a particular drug protocol and then discover that it just isn't right for you, or that your cancer doesn't respond to it.

You're going to get frustrated when you don't have the energy you expect to have when you wake up in the morning, and you're going to face setbacks along the way. But keeping your spirits up, remaining optimistic, especially in the face of discouraging evidence, means that when the right drug does come along, you'll be revved and ready to respond to it.

The scientists have a fancy expression for this kind of positive self-talk. "Neuro-linguistic programming" or NLP, was explained to me as a way of making your brain believe in something so completely that it conveys the message to the rest of your body. For example, if a child continually says to himself, "I'm no good at math," the brain hears that message and is little help when it comes to solving problems and memorizing facts.

But if instead that child is encouraged to say aloud, and to himself, "I can figure out this math," researchers suggest that the brain "gets" the message and provides the necessary pathways for this learning to take place. So perhaps what I've always called positive attitude and what others describe as having a good self-image is part of this "self-fulfilling" process. When I say or think, "I'm in good hands with my medical team, and when I do exactly what they tell me to do, I will see the best possible results from this medicine or treatment," I'm telling my brain what it needs to hear from me in order to do the best it can . . . *the best it can,* to help me heal.

❋

Joy is a gift I give myself every day. It's a quiet choice, not a noisy celebration, but it helps me remain alive to the potential of every day. I never know when I open an e-mail whether it will contain a recipe question, a request for information, or something deliciously funny and touching like this perfect piece of good advice:

EVERYTHING I NEED TO KNOW I LEARNED FROM NOAH'S ARK

1. Don't miss the boat.
2. Remember that we are all in the same boat.
3. Plan ahead. It wasn't raining when Noah built the Ark.
4. Stay fit. When you're sixty years old, someone may ask you to do something really big.

5. Don't listen to critics; just get on with the job that needs to be done.
6. Build your future on high ground.
7. For safety's sake, travel in pairs.
8. Speed isn't always an advantage. The snails were on board with the cheetahs.
9. When you're stressed, float awhile.
10. Remember, the Ark was built by amateurs; the *Titanic* by professionals.
11. No matter the storm, when you are with God, there's always a rainbow waiting.

Darkness cannot put out the Light. It can only make God brighter.

—Author Unknown

Waikiki Lemon Coconut Cream Pie

Some dishes just make you grin with pure pleasure—and what better way to show your delight! Joy is everywhere, but to find it, you sometimes have to take a bite.

❈ Serves 8

2 (4-serving) packages JELL-O sugar-free instant vanilla pudding mix

1 (4-serving) package JELL-O sugar-free lemon gelatin

1⅓ cups Carnation Nonfat Dry Milk Powder

2 cups Diet Mountain Dew

½ cup Cool Whip Free

1 teaspoon coconut extract

¼ cup flaked coconut

1 (6-ounce) Keebler graham cracker piecrust

1 tablespoon purchased graham cracker crumbs or 1 (2½-inch) graham cracker, made into crumbs

In a large bowl, combine dry pudding mixes, dry gelatin, and dry milk powder. Add Diet Mountain Dew. Mix well using a wire whisk. Blend in Cool Whip Free and coconut extract. Add 2 tablespoons coconut. Mix well to combine. Spread mixture into piecrust. In a small bowl, combine graham cracker crumbs and remaining 2 tablespoons coconut. Evenly sprinkle crumb mixture over top. Refrigerate for at least 1 hour. Cut into 8 servings.

HINT: A self-seal sandwich bag works great for crushing graham crackers.

Each serving equals:

HE: ½ Fat-Free Milk • ½ Bread • 1 Slider • 18 Optional Calories

194 Calories • 6 gm Fat • 5 gm Protein • 30 gm Carbohydrate • 549 mg Sodium • 140 mg Calcium • 1 gm Fiber

DIABETIC EXCHANGES: 1½ Starch/Carbohydrate • 1 Fat • ½ Fat-Free Milk

(from: *Cooking Healthy Across America*)

Recipes for Peace

To live in hearts we leave behind
Is not to die.
—Thomas Campbell

When we bid farewell to a loved one, the priest, minister, or rabbi often says, "Rest in peace." But for many of us, faced *now* with fighting for our lives, that kind of peace comes way too late.

In order to find peace now, and to conserve my energy for getting better, I needed to make sure that the end of my life, whenever it came, was what I wanted for myself and not what someone else chose. I spent quite a bit of time contemplating what mattered to me when I considered how I might die. And after I sorted through my feelings and shared them with my family, I felt more calm and tranquil, ready to accept whatever might come.

For some people, though, peace comes from doing exactly

the opposite of what I did—and that's a personal choice to which we are all entitled.

Peace is not just the absence of war, strain, or strife. It may be a quiet stillness that descends on each of us when we connect with the essence of our lives, or when we confront the reality that this most precious life will end someday. Peace before that final rest can be a powerful tool for emotional healing—a "recipe" for spiritual health as well as physical.

※

It didn't take a cancer diagnosis to start me thinking about what I'd like to leave behind when I finally go to sit at the Lord's table.

Perhaps it's because all my life I've treasured the legacies given to me by people I've loved and who are now gone.

I have beautiful old furniture that was my grandmother's.

I have my beloved aunt Catherine's antique chicken statues in my garden.

I serve my meals on dishes that were my mother's and my grandmothers'.

And I cherish my collection of vintage Carnival glass that was created long before I was born.

For me, living daily with precious items that carry the essence of beloved ancestors feels right. While I don't know for certain when I will leave this world, I've given a lot of thought to how I want to be remembered—and which treasured possessions of mine will find their way into the lives of the people I've loved.

Does thinking about that make you feel more sorrowful than peaceful? Then perhaps it's not the right time for you to do the same, but I'd like to share some details of my journey, which may make it easier when you're ready.

※

Ever since I began collecting cookbooks as a teenager, I've spent countless hours poring over all those best-loved recipes. I've been inspired to reinvent many of the most delicious-sounding dishes in my Healthy Exchanges style, and I've relished the privilege of losing myself in whatever down-home cooking or exotic cuisine a particular book celebrated.

But it breaks my heart to think how many cookbooks find their way to the landfill or even burned to ashes on a rubbish heap! Many of these unique collections offer so much more than fresh ideas for dinner or some new hors d'oeuvres. The church and community cookbooks provide a true picture of a place and a time that nothing else does, and those images in words and sketches should be preserved.

Well, I've been doing my part—and my best—to gather an abundance of cookbooks of all kinds for more than forty years, and while my bookshelves "runneth over," my pleasure in each volume has not diminished at all. I've got such a splendid variety, from slender booklets published nearly a hundred years ago to comb-bound or stapled fund-raising projects produced in that memorable purple color of old mimeograph machines; shelves of cookbook series from the 1950s and 1960s, when every housewife was encouraged to welcome her hubby home with a tray of *rumaki* (bacon-wrapped chicken livers!); and stacks of books on every possible kind of baked goods, from layer cakes to cookies, from marvelous muffins to fruity cobblers, buckles, bettys, and more.

Where did all these amazing books come from? I've picked them up at yard and garage sales, of course, at charity shops, and in bookstores from coast to coast as Cliff and I have traveled on book tours. Some came from complete strangers who sent me boxes in the mail because they learned of my love of cookbooks and knew that I would be a good caretaker of them. (Instead of a baby-sitter, I guess I've become a "cookbook-sitter!)

I've gotten many as gifts, received some when friends and relatives passed away, and even discovered some doozies on eBay and elsewhere online!

To me, all these books make up a unique history, not only of America and its glorious heritage as a nation of immigrants, but of the endless variety of foods prepared by the peoples of the world beyond our borders.

Now, as I contemplate the books in my collection (more than 15,000 at last count!), I feel a great sense of satisfaction knowing that I've saved them from the garbage pail and the recycling bin—and that they will be preserved after I'm gone. I've arranged to donate this legacy to a university library, where it will be available to the public for research (and for pleasure reading as well). I love the idea that they will provide reading pleasure long after I'm gone—and for many generations to come. I've set aside money in my will to provide for my books' upkeep, and I've specifically said that the books must be kept together and not sold or dispersed. (I like to say that the university gets my books when I go to Cookbook Heaven, where I hope to specialize in angel food cake!)

What has been your passion during your life so far? Are you a volunteer for the ballet, a tutor of recently arrived immigrants learning English, or perhaps a supporter of your town's community theater? You may decide to bequeath your closet full of vintage dresses to the theater (especially if your daughter doesn't want them), and you may direct that a modest bequest create a toe shoe fund or a scholarship for a local student. You don't have to be a millionaire to leave a legacy ensuring that your commitment lives on!

(You don't have to wait until you're facing serious illness or approaching your later years to think about all this. I've met people who decided to honor a new grandchild with a commemorative gift instead of yet another rocking horse. Not everyone can donate a building to the university, but all of us can leave our mark on our communities.)

※

I've always loved dishes. When I was a young girl, I felt—and still do—an enormous rush of pleasure at the sight of a beautifully set table shimmering with spotless dishes of all different styles and materials—glass, porcelain, china, pottery, and even those classic and practical dishware sets like Fiestaware!

Over the years, I've bought dishes wherever and whenever

I've found a set that pleased my eye and appealed to my heart. At this point, I'm happy (and not embarrassed!) to say that I have at least fifty sets of dishes, maybe more!

Some people may think it's foolish for any one woman to have so many sets of dishes and all the pretty accessories that go with them. For me, it's not just about owning a lot of "stuff," it's about doing what makes you happy and gives you pleasure. I don't spend a lot on my "passion"—in fact, I probably spend less on my table settings than most people spend on their hobbies. But I get so much enjoyment every three to four weeks when I transform my dining room decor and set up a whole new theme!

Some people collect stamps, and others are stockpiling the new U.S. quarters in leather-bound albums. I've known people who were passionate about scrapbooking or collecting dolls. My dishes delight me, so if I see another set of dishes on sale that appeals to me, I'm probably going to get them.

My somedays are now.

From time to time people would say to me, "What are you going to do with all those dishes?" I always answered, "Use them!" and I meant it. But finding a long-term answer to that question was something I thought about even more after I received my breast cancer diagnosis. I looked at all those stacks of dishes in my cabinets and on my shelves, and I thought, I want the people I love to have these to remember me by when I am gone.

So I made up something I called "Wishes for My Dishes." I decided that each one of my children would get to choose two sets of my dishes and that Cliff was to choose the two sets that he liked best. (I wrote this all down, so my intentions would be clear!) Then I wanted to give a set to each of my sisters, to all of my nieces and my nephews, and to save a set for every one of my grandkids.

Since that list added up to only about half of my collection, I asked that the rest go to a list of people who were very special to me. What a wonderful way to remember me, using my dishes to serve favorite recipes to family and friends!

Does it make you uncomfortable to read this or to think about how you want to handle your own legacies? All I can say is that the people who love you will want to carry out your wishes after you leave this world. And anything you can do to make it easier and clearer for them is a blessing.

My kids told me that it was a relief, as if I had taken a burden from them before they even knew they had the burden. So maybe if you think of it that way, it will be easier.

Not all of my bequests will involve material things. That's something I've always understood. Just as I have been grateful for the gifts I've inherited from my own parents and grandparents, I know that part of my legacy to the future will be the way I live on in my children and grandchildren after I'm gone.

I've often said that my son James will carry on my tradition of being the creative cook in the family. He's a talented, adventurous chef who takes the same kind of pleasure in cooking for the family as I always have. Is it just maternal pride to think he may get some of his imagination and originality from me? Wherever his ingenious nature came from, he has taken wonderful advantage of it, inventing all kinds of time-saving and labor-saving devices since he was just a teenager!

When I visit with my daughter, Becky, I get glimpses of the living legacy God has allowed me to pass along to her. She is my "caring person," the child who is so good at helping people get through difficult times. As a nurse, she worked to heal others all her adult life, but even now, in her private life as a stay-at-home mother and wife, she has succeeded in reaching out to people and leaving them in a better place.

In my youngest child, Tom, I see reflections of my own father. He's my "stat man," a brilliant thinker who is able to see the clear path through the thorniest business and financial problems. He's also the family technology whiz and has been instrumental in creating the Healthy Exchanges website and teaching his mother how to use it! But Tommy is also a creative man whose gift for writing will only get better over time. Knowing that he has inherited my talent for writing is very satisfying to this mother!

I don't know for certain about how my legacies will live on in all of my grandchildren, as many of them are still very young. But we've shared many wonderful times together, and I feel so lucky to have had (and continue to have) these occasions to share my love of everything from old-time music to planting gardens, from making pancakes to walking our land.

One of the deepest, greatest satisfactions of being a grandparent is watching these little children grow and change and become who they are meant to be. As a grandparent, I can just hug 'em and kiss 'em and love 'em—I don't have to worry about the discipline, either. I just get to be in on the fun stuff of raising them and sharing with them their family heritage.

It gives me both peace and joy to know that so much of what I am (and what my ancestors have passed on to me) will live on in the minds, hearts, and souls of the people I love best.

Have you thought about your own living legacies yet? I don't mean just a few passing thoughts, but real, deep appreciation of how you have influenced the next generations. Even if you are not a parent or grandparent, you have still touched many lives during your life—and you will leave your mark on their minds, hearts, and souls.

Aren't we lucky to have this privilege, to touch the lives of others? Even as I contemplate what life may be like for my loved ones after I'm gone, I still feel blessed to have had the life I've had!

When I was diagnosed with cancer, I was determined to put my faith and my fate in God's hands, but I also felt that I needed to make some hard decisions about how I wanted to leave this world. There are some decisions that must be made, and I could either live in denial until it was too late to decide what I wanted, or I could put my family first in an act of love that would only be tough for me.

I admit that I got very emotional thinking about the subject, because I had so much I still wanted to do. I didn't want to think about death when I was still so involved with life.

But leaving my wishes unspoken would mean putting a heavy responsibility on my family at a time when their hearts would be filled with many painful emotions. Did I love them enough to make my own choices?

I did.

I do.

❈

I've known almost from my initial diagnosis what I wanted when it came to how I was treated medically. I told Cliff and my family that (when the time comes), I want to stay here at Timber Ridge Farm for as long as I can. I know it's often possible for patients to be cared for at home, with the assistance of a local hospice and its staff. If I can have that, I told them, that's what I want.

But I went on to say that the minute my needs become more than can be handled in hospice at home, I want them to feel no hesitation to put me in a hospital or a nursing home, because I do not want to be a burden to them.

Even though my family may not look at it as a burden now, I've made it clear that there may come a time when it's a hardship to take care of me. They know that I want to stay home if I can, but if I can't, they're not to question it but just to do what's best for them *and* me.

For anyone coping with a serious illness or contemplating the end of life, there are legal papers to sign and serious questions to consider. You can find out more about "health-care proxy" forms and "power of attorney" on the Internet or from your doctor's office. Even if you find it hard to talk about what you want medically, it's good to write it down so when the time comes, your family will know exactly what you want and be able to fulfill your final wishes.

I won't deny that this is very hard to do. I cried a lot when I was talking to my family, and I cried when I was writing out the details of what I wanted when I near the end of my life. But I kept hearing this little voice inside saying, "Help your family get through this, and death will be easier to accept when the time comes." I listened to that voice, but I still cried.

Once I got the medical stuff out of the way, it was time to think about the last "event" given in my honor—and in my memory: my funeral, and the dinner that will follow.

I've talked to a lot of fellow cancer patients about planning their funerals and other end-of-life issues, and I learned that many people find it incredibly freeing, a real relief, to put down on paper and talk with their loved ones about how they would like their family and friends to gather to remember them.

I'm very detail-oriented in my life, so it's not at all surprising that I would be focused about my death. I sat down with one of my ever-present yellow legal pads and I began planning my funeral, from what I wanted to wear right down to the earrings, to what kind of music I wanted played (old-time Southern gospel music), to what I wanted at my visitation.

I sat in my favorite chair, I closed my eyes, and I imagined the scene.

I decided that as people came in and signed the guest book, I wanted each person to be handed a piece of one of my best-loved pies. People think of me as the Pie Lady, so it's only right that I leave this world by serving pie at my wake (what some call the "visitation"). I even decided that in addition to the funeral program, every person who attended would also receive a little cookbooklet of the recipes served at the dinner after my funeral.

I decided it all—who I wanted as my pallbearers, what foods I wanted at the dinner, and the songs I wanted sung at my funeral, even the color I wanted my fingernails painted— all of these little things that mattered to me. I wrote it down, I signed it and had Cliff sign it, and I gave a copy each to Becky, James, and Tommy.

My son James was very upset for a day or two. He said, "You're thinking about dying."

I said, "No, I'm not, but this is what I would like if and when that time comes, so you don't have to worry about it."

Some time later, I heard him talking to someone about how he felt. "You know, I was really upset with Mom when she did it, but it was the best thing she could have done, because now we know exactly what she wants. I'm going to do it, too, so my kids don't have to worry."

It's a liberating thing. While you're doing it, it may seem morbid, but it's freeing, for you *and* for your family members. They might have gotten some of it right if they had to decide what to do, but they wouldn't have known it all.

In fact, Cliff, who knows me very well, said, "I never would have dreamed of serving pie at your visitation, but that's what you want and that's what you're known for, so it's fine with me."

Of course, the longer I live, the more likely it is that I will choose to revise my plans—but it will be *my* decision, not something my family would have to struggle with while they are mourning. Just as we keep our wills up to date, it also makes sense to me to occasionally review with our loved ones how we want to be remembered at the end.

A while back I heard country singer Lee Ann Womack's beautiful song "Something Worth Leaving Behind." The lyrics of the song remind me that love lives on in the legacies we leave our children and in how we are remembered by those whose lives we've touched.

I don't spend a lot of time worrying about how I'll be remembered or when I'm going to die, but I feel a real sense of peace that I've discussed my final wishes with my family and written them down so they don't have to go on memory alone.

Now I can live without fear of what may happen when that time comes. Now I'll just get on with living my life as fully as I can!

I've always been a person who got an idea in my head about what I wanted to do, figured out a way to do it, and did it. Because of that aspect of my personality, I've accomplished more in my life to date than I think I ever thought I would when I was young—writing more than two dozen cookbooks, appearing on my own PBS television show, traveling the country to promote my Healthy Exchanges lifestyle. I fully believed I was living every day to the fullest.

But hearing the words *"You have cancer,"* has a definite impact on your plans for what you dreamed of doing "someday." In an instant, someday becomes a lot sooner than you expected—because you realize that you don't know how long you may have to fulfill those heartfelt ambitions and secret goals.

Of course, the truth is that none of us *really* know how long we are going to live. Life doesn't always work out the way we expect, and if we're keeping long lists of what we want to do "someday," it's more than likely that many of those future plans may never materialize. So it's important to decide what you really want in your life—and then take the steps required to make those dreams real.

It's one of those games that people sometimes play—though probably not people who are coping with cancer. They say, "If you knew you had six months to live, what would you do?" Well, when the doctor "stages" your cancer, and you hear the words *"Stage IV, with metastases,"* you know in that instant that it's no game but a real, true, serious question.

Peace comes when you figure out *your* answer.

Years ago, Erma Bombeck published a wonderful essay called "If I Had My Life to Live Over" and she got me thinking about some of the things I might have done differently if I got to rewrite the past. Wouldn't most of us change a thing or two? I'd probably have said yes more often (but no to some of the things I did more out of duty than desire). I'd have taken a few more chances, and I hope I'd have made even more time for my kids and grandkids. I'd have traveled more to faraway places, and I definitely would have had regular mammograms.

I know there are fewer years in front of me than behind me, now that I'm past sixty. Every minute has become even more precious in the months and years After Diagnosis, and I've updated my list of what I need and want to do in my lifetime, since it may be the only one I'm going to get!

※

Where did *I* begin?

By going back to where the dreams began for my family. I've often mentioned that some of my dearly loved ancestors came to this country from Ireland, and yet I had never traveled there, never had a chance to see where my family members had once lived before finding the courage to cross the Atlantic and settle here in the Midwest.

Cliff and I had talked for years about taking such a trip, especially after my two sisters decided to go about five or six years ago. They'd wanted us to go with them, but we had to reluctantly say no because I was scheduled for a book tour at the very same time.

It was so bittersweet for me. I knew almost as soon as we turned them down that we should have found a way to go. Every time I thought about missing that chance, I grew so sad.

I felt as if I'd missed something important, something I'd always regret not experiencing. Knowing that my sisters had seen where my great-grandparents set sail for America but that I had been too busy to share it with them was hard to live with. That's the thing about making choices. I loved touring to promote my books, but I was so busy, I never took the time to do some of the things I really wanted to do.

So just a few months after I was diagnosed with cancer, Cliff came to me and said, "We're not going to put it off any longer. We're going to Ireland."

That very day, we chose the dates we wanted to go and made the reservations. I'm not exaggerating when I say that it was one of the most wonderful weeks of our lives. Just to see where my great-grandparents had lived was so special. You can look all you want at photographs, go to travelogues, see movies set somewhere, but until you see it for yourself, you're just not experiencing the real thing!

It was like the closing of a circle, as if visiting my ancestors' homeland cemented an unbreakable link between their past, my present, and my children and grandchildren's future. The Irish blood that runs in us had finally had a chance to go home, and it felt so good.

If I hadn't been diagnosed with cancer, if we'd just kept going on the same breakneck pace that we thrived on, I'm pretty sure that this would have been one of those things I'd never have gotten to do. We'd have just been too busy, always booked six months in advance and never setting aside the time to do it.

But the cancer made me stop and take a deep breath, ask

myself where I was going. It turned out that part of the answer was Ireland. So we just said, We're going, these are the dates, and nothing's going to change it. I'm so glad we did. My memories of that journey "home" are something I'll cherish forever.

❊

Memories are precious.

There's nothing quite like the warmth and peace we feel when we remember all the most special times in our lives. And while as we get older, there are almost too many to recall with ease, we may be astonished at how vivid our memories are of events and people who were part of our lives twenty-five, even fifty years ago. (I feel way too young to remember anything that happened fifty years ago—but I do!)

Nowadays, I find myself thinking about the memories that my grandkids are going to have of me when I'm gone. Of course they're going to remember Grandma the cooking lady, and Grandma the gardening lady. They're also going to remember those wonderful afternoons every spring when James and Tommy bring their families over. Cliff gets our flatbed trailer out, hooks it up to the tractor, and all of us work together to take all of my garden benches, statues, and birdbaths out of storage and set them out for summer.

(We do just the reverse in late October or early November, depending on the weather. They all come and help by picking everything up and putting it away for the winter. It's a wonderful way for our family to mark the changing seasons together, and we look forward to it every spring and fall.)

Just as those are the things that my somedays are made up of, they will also be a heartwarming part of my family's memories of me in the years to come.

※

What else can we do to ensure that our most precious times and relationships are remembered? Well, every single holiday since my diagnosis, in addition to the usual gifts for birthdays and Christmas, I've sent each of my grandchildren a special holiday card just for that holiday. I always write their names and the date on the card. They get cards from me at Easter and at Thanksgiving, for Valentine's Day and Halloween, and every other holiday that Hallmark makes cards for!

I love knowing that they'll have these remembrances from me to keep after I'm gone. They'll know without a doubt that I thought about them all year long!

Postage is cheap. (Don't let the government hear me say that, because it does keep going up and up.) What I mean is, for the cost of a card or some stationery and a first-class stamp, you can tell the people you treasure just how much you care. Don't put it off—start your card-writing and letter-writing campaign today.

Another thing I'm making a real point of doing is taking lots and lots of photographs, many more than I used to. I'm trying to get as many pictures of me *with them* so that ten years from now, if I'm no longer here, they won't have forgotten what I look like. They'll have piles of photos to trigger happy memories of the times we spent together.

Man must not allow the clock and the calendar to blind him to
the fact that each moment of his life is a miracle and a mystery.
—H. G. Wells

When I first found out I had cancer, I made a list of things I regretted not doing or had put off for a faraway tomorrow. Now that I've been blessed with more time than my oncologist ever expected, and now that my cancer is in remission (at least for now), I still want every minute to count.

But here's a funny thing I've noticed: When you decide that every minute counts, you actually slow down more: to really smell the roses, to gaze into at the face of a beloved grandchild, and to listen to music that truly touches your heart. Even though time does seem to fly as you get older, you have the power to slow it down a bit—at least, for a few minutes here and there.

Are you someone who always has to be doing something or you feel as if you're being lazy? Could it be that old work ethic whispering in your ear says that the half hour you just spent sitting in your garden or chatting with a friend on the phone could have been put to better use?

I'm a great believer in working hard, and I know that belief is responsible for helping me reach many of my fondest goals. But I have also learned that there are definitely times to stop working and just breathe in the beauty of God's creations.

I mean, if we weren't meant to pause and appreciate the exquisite color of a peach blossom or the irresistible scent of an American Beauty rose or the heartwarming pleasure of a juicy strawberry, then why would God have made them?

The more I have come to understand that each day is a gift from God, the closer I feel to Him. And the more I allow myself the quiet time to appreciate the many facets of every precious moment, the more completely I feel myself warmed and filled with His love.

I've always loved the quotation from Psalms 118:24, "This is the day the Lord has made; we will rejoice and be glad in it." It resonates now for me more than ever before. Each day is a blessing, each hour a gift, and each moment a tiny treasure that can make a memory—if only we are willing to treat it as such!

God is the keeper of somedays, as He is the keeper of each and every day of our lives. So even as I pray quietly for enough "somedays" to watch my grandkids grow up, to cultivate my gardens, to share my love of good food and good health with others, and to offer my life wisdom to anyone who asks for help, I know that someday, my somedays will run out. For now, though, I will cherish those I have in every way I know.

If you can find a path with no obstacles, it probably doesn't lead anywhere.

—Frank A. Clark

Lemon Cheesecake
with Lemon Glaze

When you're digging deep emotionally to figure out what legacies of love you're going to leave behind, you need to keep up your strength. This scrumptious dessert will sustain and inspire you (I hope!).

❋ Serves 8

2 (4-serving) packages JELL-O sugar-free instant vanilla pudding mix
2 (4-serving) packages JELL-O sugar-free lemon gelatin
2 (8-ounce) packages Philadelphia fat-free cream cheese
⅔ cup Carnation Nonfat Dry Milk Powder
1¾ cups Diet Mountain Dew
1 cup Cool Whip Lite
1 (6-ounce) Keebler shortbread or graham cracker piecrust

In a small bowl, reserve 1 tablespoon dry pudding mix and 2 teaspoons dry gelatin. In a large bowl, stir cream cheese with a sturdy spoon until soft. Add dry milk powder, remaining dry pudding mix, and remaining dry gelatin to cream cheese. Stir in 1¼ cups Diet Mountain Dew. Mix well using a wire whisk. Blend in ½ cup Cool Whip Lite. Spread pudding mixture evenly into piecrust. In a small saucepan, combine reserved pudding mix and reserved gelatin with remaining ½ cup Diet Mountain Dew. Cook over medium heat, stirring constantly, until mixture starts to boil. Place saucepan on a wire rack and allow to cool 10 minutes. Drizzle mixture evenly over top of pie. Refrigerate for at least 2 hours. Cut into 8 servings. Top each serving with 1 tablespoon Cool Whip Lite.

Each serving equals:

HE: 1 Protein • ½ Bread • ¼ Fat-Free Milk • 1 Slide • 19 Optional Calories

205 Calories • 5 gm Fat • 12 gm Protein • 28 gm Carbohydrate • 830 mg Sodium • 1 gm Fiber

DIABETIC EXCHANGES: 1½ Starch • 1 Meat • 1 Fat

(from: *Cooking Healthy with a Man in Mind*)

Recipes for Hope

Hope is the thing with feathers
That perches in the soul,
And sings the tune without the words,
And never stops at all . . .
—*Emily Dickinson*

When life hands us terrible news, when the doctor utters the word *malignant,* and when pain and fear sap our spirits—*hope* remains.

Hope endures.

Hope is fueled by the knowledge that *some* people respond to the medication, *some* don't experience side effects, *some* survive for six months, a year, then five, and then—the sky's the limit!

Hope is what we have left no matter what challenge or crisis we must face. My recipe for hope is simple: Ignore the odds, silence the statistics, strengthen your faith in the Lord, and just keep tiptoeing toward the future with all you've got.

> *When the world says, "Give up,"*
> *Hope whispers, "Try it one more time."*
> —Author Unknown

Shortly after my diagnosis, one of my family members let some friends know about my illness and asked them to say a prayer for me. It was a beautiful, thoughtful thing to do. In response, she received a number of e-mails, including one from a friend offering sympathy about the fact that there was no hope. She asked, "How can she deal with living when she knows she's dying?" (I only found out about what she said because it was accidentally forwarded to me.) I wasn't offended or horrified by seeing those words in black-and-white, actually quite the opposite. It gave me a chance to say what I truly believe: It's just not as awful as you may think it is.

Yes, I had just found out I had Stage IV breast cancer, and yes, it had already spread to all the nearby lymph nodes and my bones by the time it was diagnosed. Yes, I discovered that the rare form of inflammatory breast cancer I had is one of the most aggressive kinds you can have. And yes, my doctor later admitted to me that when he first knew how bad it was, he suspected I would have no more than three to six months to live.

But "no hope"? *No way!*

Not when you put your life and your concerns in God's hands.

How could there be "no hope" when there was plenty we could do to fight the cancer? Thanks to the dedication, creativity, and years of research of scientists all over the world, there were several drug protocols that had shown encouraging results in reducing the size or slowing the growth of breast tumors. Better still, there were others on the horizon, so as long my chemo helped buy me time, I could hope that some of those might help extend my life and heal my condition.

Besides, none of us really know for sure when we're going to die, so we just have to go on living and not dwell on it. Life is infinitely more precious today than ever before, and I've chosen not to feel sorry for myself. That's why I don't want anyone else feeling sorry for me, either.

Pray for me, yes. Pity me, no.

Hope is faith holding out its hand in the dark.
—George Iles

My oncologist told me that people with cancer don't usually die from the cancer itself. Instead, they succumb because of one of three reasons: either it hits the lungs and they stop working, or it hits the kidneys and they stop working, or it just wears them down so far they can't go on.

But I don't ask my doctor about "my chances." It's just not the way that either he or I think. I don't want to listen when someone starts spouting statistics and likely rates of cure. The numbers aren't encouraging, and besides, math was never my strongest subject.

Instead, I want to hold up my hand, like Harrison Ford as Han Solo in *Star Wars* did, and simply say, "Never tell me the odds!"

That's the thing about statistics—in a very real way, they don't apply to you and here's why. Because no one in the world has exactly the same genes, the same history, the same cell wars going on in the body—and so those numbers don't include you.

Remember when they said a woman over forty had more chance of getting kidnapped by terrorists than finding a husband? It all turned out to be wrong!

Besides, plenty of women beat those odds every single day. And I'm already working toward beating the odds on this cancer, since some research suggests that ninety-five percent of Stage IV IBC patients whose cancer has metastasized won't live for five years.

I just have to live my life as if I'm in the fantastic five percent that wins this particular lottery. I need to be, and I want to be. With God's help and the prayers of friends and family, I think I can be—and you know what they say: "If you think you can, you can. If you think you can't, you're also right."

Hope is putting faith to work when doubting would be easier.
—*Author Unknown*

The Internet is such an amazing place. Besides finding wonderful support groups and inspiring essays, you often stumble upon a real-life story that touches your heart and fills you with deep emotion. That's what happened when I first read about a twelve-year-old girl from North Carolina named Hope.

Hope was in the late stages of osteosarcoma—bone cancer—when she was contacted by the Make-a-Wish Foundation. This worthy organization, which fulfills the wishes of terminally ill children, offered Hope the opportunity to have one of her dreams come true.

Hope asked them how many children were waiting to have their wishes fulfilled. The answer: 155. So Hope told them that her wish was to help raise enough money to fulfill all those wishes. The Make-a-Wish Foundation said it would need one million dollars to make them all come true. Hope's story ran on radio and television on December 19, 2003, and contributions started coming in. By December 20, they had $15,000, and by Christmas Eve, the figure had grown to $350,000. People donated money they'd saved for family vacations, and one man even donated $100,000. The owner of the Carolina Panthers football team donated some playoff tickets, which were auctioned off for $15,000. Kids emptied piggy banks and gave up their allowances, many buying special silver charms with Hope's name on them.

It was an incredible outpouring of generosity. Hope had asked that the organization hold a big party on January 16, 2004, to announce that they'd reached their goal. But as New Year's Eve approached, they were only partway there. More publicity brought more donations, and when the night finally arrived, the goal was met—more than $1.1 million raised on behalf of a young woman with an extraordinary faith in God and a truly giving heart.

Sadly, Hope didn't live to see her goal reached, but the celebration of her unique spirit goes on. In a *Charlotte Observer* article reporting on her passing, Make-a-Wish Foundation board member Chuck Coira said, "Hope allowed me to witness and experience grace. Although she is gone, I will always have Hope."

That is what I, too, will take away from this story. As long as we have faith in God, we will always have the grace of Hope.

Can I leave you with a recipe for hope?

Is such a thing possible?

I'd like to think so. I've come to believe that hope isn't just an encouraging emotion but can actually provide a structure to live by, a system to help us not only make it through the stress, fear, anger, and pain, but *prevail* over it.

When I speak to groups about my experiences, I talk about what I've come to call my "Seven Highways to Hope." I want to share them with you now. While these paths and lessons reflect my own experiences, I "hope" they may also have some useful meaning for you as you continue on your own journey.

1) Put your faith in God and your fate in His hands.

I knew from the beginning that cancer was something that I couldn't handle by myself. So I immediately turned the whole thing over to God. Each day, I pray for the strength, the courage, and the determination to live my life in a way that is pleasing to Him.

I don't pray for a cure (though of course I'd appreciate one!); rather, I pray to accept whatever it is that God wants me to accept. It's not always easy, because we humans have a tendency to want to have things go our way, but realizing that God is helping me to carry my cross makes it much more bearable.

Someday maybe I'll learn why God wanted me to experience Stage IV inflammatory breast cancer. Until then, I'll just do my part and let God take care of the rest.

2) Choose how you react to your health crisis, participate in the decision-making, and you'll be able to handle whatever comes.

Winston Churchill said, "Attitude is a little thing that makes a big difference." We can't always control what's happening to our bodies but we *can* control how we respond to what's happening each day.

Instead of dreading Fridays, my chemo day, I chose to look forward to Fridays as *my day*. After I get my treatment, I spend the rest of the afternoon doing whatever I choose.

By combining my treatment with pleasurable activities, I've moved my Friday focus from treating my cancer to enjoying how this change in my schedule has also changed my life for the better. I can face my chemo more positively because I know the rest of the day is mine to enjoy in whatever way I choose.

3) Celebrate all the little things that make life good, and take time to cherish the people you love.

It may be an old cliché, but you really do start to appreciate every sunrise you're blessed to witness. You really do take the time to smell the roses. You cherish the hugs and kisses your grandchildren shower on you. You delight in catching up on what's going on with your loved ones while chatting with them on the phone. And you don't get upset when whatever plans you have for the day are changed because of circumstances beyond your control. You simply are thankful for the chance to live another day.

This isn't to say that you'll need to give up your career dreams or long-held ambitions. This is about what *you value,* and for each of us, that will vary greatly. You may choose to grow your business or pursue a new occupation, perhaps even one inspired by your effort to cope with your illness. But I believe you'll find that family and friends become much, much more important to you.

How does that old quote go? "When you're finally on your deathbed, are you going to wish you'd worked more, or spent more time with the people you love?" Ain't it the truth!

4) *Surround yourself with people who will stick by you in good times and bad.*

If you're married, you'll soon learn how well you chose way back when, especially if you followed your heart instead of your head! Cliff and I have been married for a quarter of a century now, a second marriage for both of us, and it's clear that we're in it for the long run. But tough times test any marriage, and it's been an eye-opener to see how my husband was willing and able to adapt.

What if you're single, or divorced, or widowed? Who's going to be there for you? That's an important question to answer, and it's up to you to line up your team of "go-to" friends and relatives. A friend in New York City told me about getting a phone call from an elderly neighbor at 3 A.M. and helping him get to the emergency room when he needed it. "He put me on his 'contact in case of emergency' card, not his brother or sister in Ohio," she said. "Here, for many of us, our friends are our family."

Even if you feel that your loved ones have already seen you at your worst, you may be unprepared for how much you'll need to depend on them when you're desperately ill or emotionally shaken. In the middle of the night, or when you're shivering with fever, you need to know you can count on them.

So you can't settle for lightweights. It takes real guts to be a friend through thick and thin—and you may already know that because you've been there for someone else.

If you feel that you've let the kind of friends you need slip away, it's *not too late!* Talk to them honestly, reconnect solidly, and always let them know how much you value their commitment to helping you through your journey of survival.

5) *Get as many opinions as you want and need—then commit to your medical team and use all its resources.*

I consider myself lucky that I found what has been for me the ideal combination: great medical treatment not far from home and an unshakable faith in God to see me through. I found a great oncologist in a clinic right here in the Quad Cities, and together we map out my treatments. My doctor has treated me like a partner in this process (which I need to be), and has shared with me what I can expect from whatever protocol I'm on. I've learned that he likes to think in six-month chunks, and while I'm doing my best to respond to the treatments, he's researching new protocols that just might give me another six months when and if this medication has run its course.

I was lucky to find what I needed "in my own backyard," which greatly increased my quality of life. I know not everyone can do that, and it has meant a lot to me. Because it's less than thirty minutes from my front door to my oncology clinic, I'm not spending hours on the road and days away from home to get my treatment.

I believe that one of the reasons I've done so well is that I've made a genuine commitment: to the treatments I'm getting and to a medical team I've entrusted with my life. And because the nurses and doctors sense that I'm working with them one hundred percent, I feel that they're giving me their best efforts, too.

6) *Save your strength for what you value most.*

I've had to learn my own physical limitations during my treatment for cancer, and now I don't try to do more than I can or I should. Just as emergency workers "triage" patients so the ones that need the most immediate attention get it first, I've started performing triage on my own life.

If it's a project that involves my family (especially my grandchildren), my gardens, or my Healthy Exchanges endeavors, then I will find the strength and energy to do it.

If it doesn't, then maybe I will—and maybe I won't.

I've learned to say "No" with a smile. I'm no longer embarrassed to say it, and that represents a real change for me. While I will usually conserve my strength enough to go to my grandchildren's activities (school plays, open houses, or soccer games) or to programs at my church, I no longer feel I have to be involved in every worthy civic event or activity that's announced.

It's the same with housework. I've always taken pride in my tidy home, but now I don't have to do it all. I no longer care if there are enough dust bunnies gathered under my bed to hold a convention!

And while I still love creating my "common folk" healthy

recipes and writing my newsletters, magazine articles, and cookbooks, I no longer attend all the conventions and meetings of the various business organizations I belong to.

To make sure you have the energy to do what you truly care about, you're going to have to do *less*. But as they say, "Less is more." What I choose to do means more to me, and what I skip isn't missed much.

You may also need more rest—I know I do. My chemo protocol tends to cause my blood counts to go down, which in turn makes me very tired. I've learned not to feel guilty when I take a thirty-minute nap in the afternoon. In fact, I almost look forward to the luxury of it now!

7) Live now, live fully, so you'll have as few regrets as possible when you reach the end of your life—no matter when that may be.

Life is too short.

Sometimes, it's shorter than we ever thought it would be. So it's more important than ever to live life on your own terms and not let memorable experiences and precious moments elude your grasp!

If you've always wanted to travel, and you promised yourself you'd do it *someday,* maybe your someday is now.

If you've always wanted to learn to knit, or golf, or draw, or create stained glass windows, what are you waiting for?

If you've been thinking about redecorating your house, but

you haven't because you thought it was an unnecessary expense, why not do it now—while you can still enjoy it?

I always loved the quotation that reads, "When we look back on our lives, we regret more what we didn't do than what we did." The French singer Edith Piaf was famous for singing *"Je Ne Regrette Rien,"* or for those of us who didn't take French in school, "I Regret Nothing."

What a way to go!

※

The singer-actor Jon Bon Jovi has written: "Map out your future but do it in pencil." That's how I look at my life now. I'm always making plans, but I know that every moment is precious. And who was it who said "None of us get out of here alive"? He or she was right!

In the meantime, I'm living my life and making every minute count. This book isn't the end of my journey but the beginning of the rest of my life. I don't know what lies ahead, but I'm trusting in God to show me the way!

A bend in the road is not the end of the road . . . unless you fail to make the turn.

—Author Unknown

Luscious Lemon Meringue Pie

How can you not feel optimistic when you've got a gorgeous piece of healthy pie in front of you? Some desserts remind you that life, with all its struggles, is still a gift from God!

❃ Serves 8

1 refrigerated unbaked 9-inch pie-crust
2 cups Splenda Granular
6 tablespoons cornstarch
1¾ cups diet lemon-lime soda pop
2 egg yolks
2 tablespoons + 2 teaspoons reduced-calorie margarine
½ cup lemon juice
4 to 6 drops yellow food coloring
6 egg whites
½ teaspoon vanilla extract

Preheat oven to 425 degrees. Place piecrust in a 9-inch pie plate. Flute edges and prick bottom and sides with tines of a fork. Bake for 8 to 10 minutes or until lightly browned. Place pie plate on a wire rack and allow to cool completely. Lower oven temperature to 350 degrees. Meanwhile, in a medium saucepan, combine 1½ cups Splenda and cornstarch. Gradually stir in soda pop. Cook over medium-high heat until mixture thickens and starts to boil, stirring constantly. Lower heat and simmer for 2 minutes. Remove from heat. Place egg yolks in a large bowl. Stir 1 cup of hot filling mixture into yolks. Stir yolk mixture into mixture in saucepan. Continue cooking for 2 minutes or until mixture comes to a boil, stirring constantly. Remove from heat. Add margarine, lemon juice, and food coloring. Mix well to combine. Pour hot mixture into cooled piecrust. In a large bowl, beat egg whites with an electric mixer until soft peaks form. Add remaining ½ cup Splenda and vanilla extract. Continue beating until stiff peaks form. Spread meringue mixture evenly over filling mixture, being sure to seal to edges of piecrust. Bake for 12 to 14 minutes until meringue starts to turn golden brown. Place pie plate on a wire rack and let set for 45 minutes. Refrigerate for at least 2 hours. Cut into 8 servings.

HINTS: (1) Egg whites beat best at room temperature. (2) Meringue pie cuts easily if you dip a sharp knife in warm water before slicing.

Each serving equals:

HE: 1 Bread, • 1 Fat • ½ Protein • ½ Slider • 7 Optional Calories

---

210 Calories • 10 gm Fat • 4 gm Protein • 26 gm Carbohydrate • 194 mg Sodium • 9 mg Calcium • 1 gm Fiber

---

DIABETIC EXCHANGES: 1½ Starch/Carbohydrate • 1 Fat • ½ Meat

(from: *Cooking Healthy with Splenda*)

Resources

I've discovered that not having information to answer my questions and not finding support when I really need to talk about my illness can produce fear, confusion, and tremendous isolation. So I wanted to offer a Resources section in this book that shares some of the most useful websites and information I've found helpful on my cancer journey.

Remember, though, these are the ones that worked for me. If you're coping with a different kind of cancer or another serious disease, there are sites just for you. And if you have questions or concerns about almost anything, try putting a phrase like "cancer nutrition" or "pain in joints" in quotes when using an Internet search engine, such as Google, to find what you need—it usually works!

(I've also included a little section about inflammatory breast cancer, a rare form of breast cancer that has given me such an education in the past few years, and one about Herceptin®, the truly remarkable drug that has been instrumental in saving the lives of many women with breast cancer.)

⁘

Most of us have read the pamphlets at the doctor's office, and we've been encouraged to pay attention to changes in our breasts. A majority of women have wisely committed to having an annual breast exam by their physicians, and most also get regular mammograms, to help diagnose cancerous tumors that are too small or inaccessible to be felt by the doctor's hands or your own.

But as good as mammograms are, *they're not infallible.* And as helpful as an experienced physician's manipulation of your breast tissue is in discovering medical concerns, it's not foolproof, either. Sometimes, even when you do everything "right," you still find out you have cancer.

First, not all breast cancer begins with a lump. It's important to remember that, so that you don't dismiss physical changes in your breast but instead get them checked out. Many, even most, of the lumps that women find in their breasts are benign (meaning they're not cancerous, they don't affect nearby tissue, they don't spread, and they're usually not dangerous or life-threatening), and that's important to know as well. If you feel something different or strange, don't automatically assume you've got cancer, but also don't talk yourself out of seeing your doctor to find out for certain if a lump is malignant or not. Time is precious when it comes to treating cancer, so ask for an urgent appointment if you're concerned.

So What Is Inflammatory Breast Cancer, Anyway?

I always liked feeling unique but let me tell you, if there's one area in life where you'd be better off not being so special, it's when it comes to certain cancer diagnoses. Here's how it was explained to me: If there are one hundred women with breast cancer in any given room, about ninety-six of them would have what I would call "normal breast cancer." That is, a malignant lump found in the breast. Depending on the size of the tumor and whether it's spread at the time of diagnosis, it would be classified somewhere between Stage IA and Stage IV.

Four out of one hundred breast cancer patients—the remaining four women in the room—would be diagnosed with inflammatory breast cancer. IBC patients are generally classified at Stage IIIB once it's discovered, or even Stage IV if the cancer has metastasized (traveled elsewhere in the body).

Three out of every four women with inflammatory breast cancer will be deemed HER2 NEU negative. This means that they test negative for a particular body protein. Their cancer is still very serious and potentially deadly, but it's not quite as aggressive as that affecting the remaining one of four women who tests positive for the protein, whose cancer most likely will be one of the most aggressive breast cancers ever seen.

Of course, I'm that woman.

As soon as I got my diagnosis, I went to the Internet to find out more. They say that a little knowledge can be dangerous, but as you're the one coping with cancer, you owe it to yourself to find out as much as you can. That can mean facing the worst that could happen, but it also means finding every last pocket of hope and encouragement, every possible weapon in your fight to survive this illness.

Here's some of what I learned.

Inflammatory breast cancer is considered an uncommon but very aggressive type of breast cancer that is already deemed Stage IIIB once it's diagnosed. The most significant feature of inflammatory breast cancer is redness involving all or part of the breast. In this type of breast cancer, breast cancer cells block the lymph vessels in the skin of the breast. This blockage may cause the breast to become red, swollen, and warm to the touch. The skin of the breast may also appear pink, purple, or bruised, and it may appear pitted, like the skin of an orange (called *peau d'orange*). Part or all of the breast may be puffy, enlarged, and hard. There may also be ridges, welts, or a rash of hives on the breast.

These changes can often occur quickly, over a period of days or weeks. Another sign of this type of breast cancer can be swollen lymph nodes under the arm, above the collarbone, or in both locations. Often, no tumor can be felt, and it may not be seen on a mammogram, either.

Almost 50 percent of the time, there may be a mass you can feel or see in the breast, in addition to the redness and swelling of the breast and skin. But an infection of the breast is a much more common reason for swelling and redness of the breast— which is why doctors usually think of that first. If you are breast-feeding, for instance, infection is not unusual. But with antibiotic treatment, the infection will clear up quickly. Inflammatory breast cancer does not respond to antibiotics, and even a biopsy may not show that anything is seriously wrong. But if the redness and swelling continue to grow worse, a woman must return to the doctor for additional tests.

The diagnosis of inflammatory breast cancer is generally made by a skilled physical examination, but your physician will confirm it with additional biopsies. Alas, not every doctor has ever seen it and so the condition can be confusing.

In most cases, once a diagnosis of IBC is made, treatment will generally mean chemotherapy at first, followed by surgery and radiation. Other options including anti-estrogen medications as well as Herceptin® (Trastuzumab) therapy may also have a role. What kind of treatment you get depends on your unique situation, but it's good to be aware of possible courses of treatment.

Inflammatory breast cancer can affect anyone, but I was surprised to discover that a large number of cases involve either young women in their twenties and thirties just having children or nursing their babies, or the flip side of that coin, older women in their fifties who have recently passed through menopause.

What Happens When You Find Out You Have Cancer?

Cancers of the breast are as varied as the women, and more rarely men, who are diagnosed with them. Your doctors will try to analyze what your cancer is like, asking questions such as how big is the tumor, how fast is it growing, how is it affecting the tissues around it?

You'll be tested and retested, examined and re-examined. Your medical team will be trying to find out the *stage* of your cancer—is it contained (encapsulated) or is it spreading, invading other parts of your body? They'll also need to find out if any lymph nodes are involved and if so, how many. (Why? Because what travels through the lymphatic system of your body carries cells with it, and when cancer cells travel, they may allow a cancer of the breast to spread to your organs and bones.)

These tests will make it possible for your doctors to decide on a course of treatment they feel will attack the cancer and strengthen your body's ability to fight it off. Ask questions, make sure you understand what they're telling, and take notes so you can refer to them later and discuss them with family or friends if you choose. (I was lucky in that I had my sisters and Cliff in the room when I got my diagnosis, so they were able to help me remember what the doctors said.)

I learned that inflammatory breast cancer grows rapidly and that the cancer cells often spread to other parts of the body. Most women with an IBC diagnosis receive two kinds of treatment: *local* treatment to remove or destroy the cancer in the breast, and *systemic* treatment (throughout the system) to kill or at least control cancer cells that may have spread to other parts of the body. Local treatment affects only cells in the tumor and the area close to it; systemic treatment affects cells throughout the body.

While every case is different, here's what happens in many cases: The doctor will choose to do *surgery* as the local treatment, often coupled with *radiation therapy* to the breast and underarm. The systemic treatment is typically *chemotherapy* (anticancer drugs) or *hormonal therapy* (drugs that interfere with the effects of estrogen, the female hormone), or *both*. Some women also may have what's called *biological therapy,* which stimulates the immune system to fight the cancer.

The good news: The arsenal of weapons against this disease continues to grow. Research is ongoing to learn about different combinations of treatments (referred to as new protocols). Scientists hope that blending the latest chemotherapy drugs with hormonal therapy and biological therapy will help the patients diagnosed with IBC today, tomorrow, and for years to come.

You can find the latest information about ongoing clinical trials (research studies) from the clinical trials page of the National Cancer Institute's (NCI) website at http://cancer.gov/clinical_trials on the Internet.

Cancer Information, Treatment, and Support

Inflammatory Breast Cancer Support
www.ibcsupport.org

IBC Research Organization
www.ibcresearch.org

Inflammatory Breast Cancer Memorial
www.ibcmemorial.org

Inflammatory Breast Cancer Facts (National Cancer Institute)
http://cis.nci.nih.gov/fact/6_2.htm

Information about Herceptin®
www.herceptin.com

Cancer Information Service
Toll-free: 1-800-4-CANCER (1-800-422-6237)
TTY (for deaf and hard-of-hearing callers): 1-800-332-8615

National Cancer Institute Online
www.nci.nih.gov

American Cancer Society
1-800-ACS-2345
www.cancer.org

Breastcancer.org
www.breastcancer.org

Breast Cancer Fund
1-415-346-8223
www.breastcancerfund.org

Cancer Care, Inc.
1-800-813-HOPE
www.cancercare.org

National Alliance of Breast Cancer Organizations (NABCO)
1-888-80-NABCO
www.nabco.org

National Breast Cancer Coalition
1-202-296-7477
www.natlbcc.org

Susan G. Komen Breast Cancer Foundation, Inc.
1-800-IM AWARE
www.komen.org

Y-ME National Breast Cancer Organization
1-800-221-2141 (24-hour hotline)/1-800-986-9505 (Spanish)
www.y-me.org

BCMets (for people with breast cancer metastases)
www.bcmets.org

HER2 Support
http://www.her2support.org/
for those who are HER2 "protein-positive"

Nutrition

The American Institute for Cancer Research (AICR) offers a Nutrition Hotline (1-800-843-8114) 9 A.M. to 5 P.M., E.T., Monday to Friday. This free service allows you to ask questions about nutrition, diet, and cancer. A registered dietitian will return your call, usually within 48 hours. According to their website, AICR is the only major cancer charity focusing exclusively on the link between diet, nutrition, and cancer. The Institute is responsible for providing educational programs that help millions of Americans make nutritional changes to lower their cancer risk. AICR also supports cutting-edge research in cancer prevention and treatment at universities, hospitals, and research centers across the United States. Visit www.aicr.org.

Herceptin®

Because Herceptin has been such an important part of my treatment for inflammatory breast cancer, I wanted to share some information about this "miracle" drug. This information is from the Herceptin website, courtesy of Genentech Inc.

Herceptin® (Trastuzumab) is a unique biologic therapy for women with HER2-positive metastatic breast cancer. This monoclonal antibody therapy differs from traditional treatments, such as chemotherapy and hormone-blocking therapy. Herceptin works by specifically targeting tumor cells that overexpress the HER2 protein.

Herceptin is FDA-approved for first-line use in combination with Paclitaxel for the treatment of HER2 protein overexpressing metastatic breast cancer. Therapy varies from patient to patient. Clinical trials have shown that Herceptin administered either in combination with chemotherapy or alone may noticeably reduce tumor size, increase median time to disease progression, and increase one-year survival rates.

While chemotherapy can affect healthy cells as well as cancerous cells, Herceptin targets mostly tumor cells that overexpress the HER2 protein. Patients who are given Herceptin alone may be less likely to experience the side effects typical of other types of treatments, such as hair loss, fatigue, or a decline in certain blood counts. The most common side effects associated with Herceptin have been infusion-related. However, other side effects have occurred.

What is a monoclonal antibody?

An antibody is a protein made by the body's own natural immune system. They are directed against foreign and infectious agents, called antigens. Monoclonal antibodies engineered through biotechnology are produced to provide specific antitumor action within the human body.

How does Herceptin work?

Monoclonal antibody therapy works in a different way than standard cancer therapy, such as chemotherapy or hormone therapies. Herceptin® (Trastuzumab) is believed to function in three different ways:

1) *Blocking tumor cell growth.* Herceptin binds to the HER2 proteins (receptors) on the tumor cell surface. The HER2 proteins, with Herceptin attached, are pulled back into the cell. When the HER2 proteins are no longer on the cell surface, they can no longer tell the cell to grow and divide.

2) *Signaling of the immune system.* Herceptin attaches to the HER2 proteins (receptors) on a tumor cell. Then certain immune system cells, called natural killer (NK) cells, are attracted to Herceptin. The NK cells detect that the cell is abnormal, and attach to Herceptin. Finally, the NK cells kill the tumor cell.

3) *Working with chemotherapy.* Herceptin and chemotherapy work in different ways, but when given together, the two drugs can form a partnership. For example, when Herceptin is used with chemotherapy that attacks and damages the DNA in the cell nucleus of tumors, Herceptin stops the cells from repairing themselves. Because these damaged cells cannot heal, they die. This slows the growth of tumors.

What is HER2?

HER2 stands for human epidermal growth factor receptor 2. HER2 is a gene that helps control how cells grow, divide, and repair themselves. The HER2 gene directs the production of special proteins, called HER2 receptors. About one out of four breast cancers has too many copies of the HER2 gene or too many receptors.

What does it mean to be HER2-positive?

Each healthy breast cell contains two copies of the HER2 gene, which contribute to normal cell function. If something goes wrong in our bodies, a change can occur that causes too many copies of a certain gene to appear. This is referred to as gene amplification. If extra copies of the HER2 gene appear in a cell, the gene can cause too many HER2 proteins, or receptors, to appear on the cell surface. This is referred to as HER2 protein overexpression. Patients who are considered HER2-positive have HER2 gene amplification or HER2 protein overexpression. Cancers with too many copies of the HER2 gene or too many HER2 receptors tend to grow fast. They are also associated with an increased risk of spread.

Why should you know your HER2 status?

HER2 protein overexpression or gene amplification affects about 25 percent of breast cancer patients and results in a more aggressive form of the disease. Patients with HER2 protein overexpression or gene amplification may also experience earlier disease reappearance, and the disease may not be as responsive to standard therapies. The results of an HER2 test can give you and your doctor insights into your disease and help you make more informed decisions about your treatment.

How do you get a HER2 test?

Testing is done on tumor tissue and should ideally be performed at the time of diagnosis. Patients who want their HER2 status checked should ask their physician to have testing done at the time of biopsy or surgery, or on their stored tumor tissue. Your doctor will send your tumor block, or tissue, to a pathology lab for further evaluation.

What kind of testing for HER2 is available?

The FDA has approved two tests, IHC (DAKO HercepTest®) and FISH (Vysis Path Vysion®), for the selection of patients for Herceptin® (Trastuzumab). Find out your test results and which test was performed. This is important. Breast cancers that test IHC "3+" or FISH "positive" should respond well to Herceptin®.

1) ImmunoHistoChemistry (IHC): To determine if your cancer is HER2-positive the IHC test is used to measure

HER2 protein (also called HER2 receptor) overexpression in the tumor sample. When large quantities of HER2 protein are produced, or overexpressed, the tumor cells can grow and divide more quickly. The results of HercepTest® can be reported as 0, 1+, 2+, or 3+. If the result is 3+, your cancer is considered HER2-positive. If the result is 2+, your cancer is borderline, and you can and should ask to have the tissue tested with the FISH test. If the result is 0 or 1+, your cancer is considered HER2-negative, and your doctor may or may not choose to retest with FISH.

2) Fluorescence In Situ Hybridization (FISH): The FISH test can be used to determine your HER2 status. It uses fluorescent probes to "paint" the HER2 genes in a tumor cell, to see if the number of gene copies is normal or not. A normal cell has two copies of the HER2 gene. If a FISH test detects more than two copies of the HER2 gene, it means that the cell is abnormal and is HER2-positive. This abnormality is also referred to as HER2 gene amplification. The results of the FISH test can be reported as "positive" or "negative."

Your doctor may choose to do IHC, FISH, or both tests. Ask your doctor if you have more questions about HER2 testing.

What if you have already had a biopsy, but do not know if you have been screened for HER2?

Pathology labs may keep biopsy tissue for a number of years, so your tissue can potentially be evaluated for HER2 protein overexpression or gene amplification with a HER2 test. Just ask your doctor to contact the facility where your sample was taken in order to find out whether the HER2 test has been performed. If it has not, your doctor can request that the test be performed on the stored tissue sample, commonly called archived tissue. A FISH test may be preferred when testing a stored tissue sample.

What if your biopsy is no longer being stored?

If you are told that your tissue is no longer being stored and you have a recurrence of the cancer, it may be possible for your physician to perform a new biopsy of an area where the tumor has grown back. For more information about the options available to you, be sure to ask your doctor.

If you have a positive HER2 status, you may be a candidate for Herceptin therapy. Remember, no matter what your HER2 status is, it is important to thoroughly discuss all your treatment options with your oncologist, as well as your family members and support groups.

Genentech, the makers of Herceptin®, offers a program for patients and their family members called Finding Your Way. It's designed to educate women and their families about breast cancer and also to promote awareness about breast cancer, and about the latest testing and treatment options. If you'd like to order the program, you may call Genentech at 1-800-818-9188 or go to their website to order it online: http://www.herceptin.com; follow the link to Patient and Caregiver.

You may also find copies of this material in your doctor's office or at the hospital where you receive treatment.

As this book goes to press in early summer 2005, the cancer came back for the fourth time, and I'm now on my seventh chemo protocol. What the previous six drugs couldn't do, this one finally did. I lost my hair in a matter of days, and now I'm wearing that wig I bought more than three years ago when I was first diagnosed.

After having a really good cry, I decided I would rather see my grandchildren grow than my hair, and I don't begrudge one moment of having to wear that curly blond wig. Besides, all the money I'm saving at the hairdresser's, I'm now spending on more flowers and shrubs for my gardens—and on my grandkids, of course!

I expect that there will be plenty more curves in the road of my cancer journey, and I'm determined to meet each of them with a sense of humor and a feeling of gratitude for every day God grants me. None of us knows how our lives will unfold, but living with cancer makes every minute more precious.

I want to hear from you . . .

Now that I've shared my cancer journey, I'd like to know how yours is going, so please feel free to contact me by mail, fax, or e-mail. We're in this together!

> Write: JoAnna M. Lund
>   c/o Healthy Exchanges, Inc.
>   P.O. Box 80
>   DeWitt, IA 52742-0080
> Fax: 1-563-659-2126 or contact me via
> E-mail: HealthyJo@aol.com

Visit my Healthy Exchanges Internet website at: http://www.healthyexchanges.com